This book is for you if

- You have tried every diet go

- You have persistent, negative thoughts around your health and weight

- You struggle with confidence, self-esteem and happiness

- You need motivation and practical hints and tips that fit in to your busy lifestyle

- You are 'time-poor' – a new parent, a stressed professional, a full-time carer, or someone trying to balance multiple demands on their time

- You want to get a clear understanding of what's holding you back and a clear plan of how to fit weight loss and a healthy lifestyle in your busy life.

Words of praise

"As a healthcare professional, scientist and someone who has always struggled with weight, I find Anne's book and 5 steps balanced, factual and empathetic without being preachy. This book is a journey of self-esteem, acceptance and understanding the science behind leading a healthy lifestyle.

I promise that you will not put it down for a second and will be galvanised to take action and responsibility for your state of being."
Dr Syeda Saleha Hassan
Health-Care Professional

—

"This is a fantastic book for anyone who wants to take the power back that they have to transform their mind and body. It's carefully thought out and well put together.

Anne is someone who I've known for many years. She an expert in the science of change and has been able to get amazing results with her clients. She's an absolutely incredible professional. This book will help people get rid of the confusion, get rid of all the myths and get people the practical information that they need to go about transforming their body.

This book is a must-read for people who want to seize back ownership of their health, their wellbeing and wanting to live an exceptional life."
Pete Cohen
Best-selling Author, Life-coach and Keynote Speaker

"From reading the first words to the last in Anne's book, it is easy to see and feel that she has a clear understanding of her field of expertise - weight loss and becoming confident, happy and fulfilled.

Anne's conversational style makes the book flow and is simple to read, understand and remember, and is highly motivational. Some key parts will resonate immensely with her readers. I, for one, am looking forward to working through Anne's book as I have realised that there are elements of the book that I really have to address.

Her WHY exercise is such a deep coaching strategy. When the 'aha' moment is realised and the WHY found and understood, then success is so much easier to achieve."
Brenda Dempsey
The Spirited Leader - Master Coach, International Best-selling Author, Speaker

—

"If you're looking for an approach that will adapt to your life in all its complexity and that works for you, no matter how complex your life is, then Anne's book is the right one for you. It is a pleasure to read and is full of stories from clients she worked with over the years and how she dealt with their issues in a professional and compassionate way. In this book you will clarify why you want to lose weight, you will work on your mindset, you will learn how to plan and create helpful habits, learn about nutrition, physical activity and how to deal with stress and sleep for optimal weight loss. It's a very complete, yet adaptable method. I certainly recommend it."
Brigitte Lipschutz PhD
Coach and Trainer

"I needed this book a long time ago! Actually - anyone who has struggled with their health and wellbeing and tried numerous diets, eating plans and exercise regimes as I have - NEEDS this book NOW! I have read numerous books over the years as I searched for that elusive 'miracle' to help me finally feel better, eat better, sleep better and ultimately look better. Just a heads up…there is NO miracle! YOU make the choices and YOU handle the consequences of all the wellbeing choices you make!

Anne's book and her simple but powerful five steps approach is the answer for me, and only now I am confident to run my own race with my health and fitness. I have developed habits that make me happy and feel good and that fit in with my life and I know I will keep them for life. I have learned that adopting a healthy and active lifestyle should not be a 'quick fix' but something that you create for yourself and that becomes part of your day, week, month, year and life and is unlikely to be the same as anyone else's.

If you love how you feel when you are engaged with your habits around health, nutrition and wellbeing then you will continue to do whatever it is that makes you feel so good because you will remember the emotion you felt when you did whatever it was - whether that is drinking more water, walking every day, preparing fresh, home-cooked food or running 5K. I have done this with the help of Anne's brilliantly written, clear and coherent book and I cannot recommend it highly enough. It's a book and an approach that is refreshing and insightful and useful for everyone, but as someone who has found the menopause particularly challenging, it has really hit the spot. Thank you Anne!"

Sarah Adams
Journalist, Lecturer and Author of The Life Edit

"Anne's 5 steps are easy to read and understand with real life examples to associate with each step. It's good to know how others have worked through their obstacles and achieved success through doing the work. I love that she explains there's no magic click of the fingers, it's a process, and that finding your "Why" (Part 2 of the book) will be the continual driver to take actions that create the change you want to see and feel."

Nikki Love
Adventure Runner

—

"Anne's book is packed full of simple, practical tips in a structure that guides you effortlessly and effectively through a clear process. With Anne's years of experience and knowledge, the tools in this book will help you achieve your goals, and feel happier for life. I've known Anne for years and she is a supportive, knowledgeable and caring coach, which is evident in her writing and the process, which is easy and accessible. Jump in, read and start taking action today..."

Kim Ingleby
Award-winning Mind Body Coach, TEDx Speaker & Author

5 Simple Steps to Releasing the Real You

How to become Confident, Happy and Fulfilled

Georgeto,
Be healthy
Be happy
Thrive!

Anne

Anne Iarchy

Published by
Filament Publishing Ltd
16, Croydon Road, Waddon, Croydon,
Surrey, CR0 4PA, United Kingdom
Telephone +44 (0)20 8688 2598
Fax +44 (0)20 7183 7186
info@filamentpublishing.com
www.filamentpublishing.com

© Anne Iarchy 2020

The right of Anne Iarchy to be identified as the author of this work
has been asserted by her in accordance with the
Designs and Copyright Act 1988.

ISBN 978-1-913192-70-9

Printed by 4Edge

Contents

Introduction

My name is Anne, and I'm a Haribo addict, in remission…

I was never a slim child. On top of the healthy meals we ate at home, I spent a chunk of my pocket money on sweets and bakery goods. In primary school, I was very active. I loved sports and exercise. Being so active meant that the full damage of my sweet tooth wasn't properly visible.

From high school onwards, my activity levels dropped. After university, I started my career in the hi-tech industry. Regular hours weren't really part of my life for many years, and frequent work travel made adopting a routine nearly impossible. Airport, aeroplane, train, hotel and restaurant food were the norm, in addition to client entertainment with some drinks to top it off. Nights were cut short due to travel, which led to me being perpetually tired. A great excuse to stop exercising, except for my weekend golf games when I was at home.

My fridge at home was always empty. After all, what's the point of coming home to rotten fruit and vegetables, and lumpy milk? Takeaways when home or just eating out with friends was the easy option. To combat the tiredness, I filled up on Haribos for quick energy. Nurofen kept the headaches at bay and helped me to relax.

As you can imagine, that lifestyle wasn't conducive to a healthy weight, which crept up slowly but surely. I tried many diets during those years, but as most were so restrictive, they were impossible to follow long-term with my lifestyle. Over the years, I spent lots of money on gym memberships I rarely used, even with good intentions to go when I wasn't travelling.

I kept on asking the personal trainers for advice on how I could lose weight with my hectic, unstructured life. Unfortunately, none managed to come up with a plan. For them, it was all or nothing.

One day, I signed up once more at another local gym and was offered five sessions with one of their personal trainers to get me kick-started. During our chat, she asked me about my goals, my exercise background, and my eating habits. I explained to her that I was leading a hectic lifestyle including lots of travel, and very proudly, I mentioned that the last few months I had really tried to be "good" and reduced a bit of the sweet quantity.

I was shocked by her answer: "Unless you're going to take it seriously and be fully committed, it's just not good enough." I didn't even know how to respond and switched off for the rest of our chat.

After our session, I ran straight to the shops to buy a few bags of Haribos… I never saw her again for the other four sessions.

I wasn't happy in myself, my confidence was low, and I didn't like what I saw in the mirror or in pictures.

On a "fun" afternoon out with work, I fell and tore the ligaments in my knee. I have always been interested in the human body and how it works. (My dad still thinks I would have made a terrific doctor.) I was intrigued by the rehab process – how the muscles worked, and how to strengthen certain muscles that would take over the function of my ligaments.

I eventually looked for a personal training course that I could combine with my more than full-time job. Although I completed the course in 2007, it was only at the start of 2010, after some management changes in the company I worked for, that I made my big career change.

I wanted to help busy people just like me to lose weight, gain confidence and feel happy within themselves.

Quite quickly I realised that, as a regular personal trainer, I would only get my clients very limited results, just as I'd got when I used personal trainers. I had to offer a more complete package, so I added nutrition to the mix, together with training. My clients started to get better results.

However, many still didn't keep to their eating plans for the usual reasons/ excuses. There was more to weight loss than just "eat less, move more". And that although, at the end of the day, being in calorie deficit is what is going to provide weight loss, the way to get to this is not as straightforward as diets describe it to be. It's never just your diet.

I looked at habits, mindset, sleep and stress, which were the recurring issues my clients brought up as reasons why they didn't stick to their plans. And over the past 10 years, I have developed a 5-step system that gives my client consistent long-term results. My hope is that, when applying the system, you as a reader of this book will get the results you always wanted.

If you've been struggling with your weight, and have tried many diets, or potentially the same diet over and over again, without long-term results, then this book is for you.

If you've been struggling to juggle the pressures of life, work, family, social life, hobbies, and anything else that is keeping you busy, and use those as a reason/excuse for your struggle with weight, then this book is for you.

If you feel that the lack of willpower and/or self-discipline is what is holding you back from achieving your weight loss goal, then this book is for you.

If you are ready to be open to new ideas, and to explore new methods, while forgetting everything you've ever learned on previous attempts, then this book is for you.

This book will give you the tools to achieve weight loss for life and become totally awesome! You will finally understand that there is much more to weight loss than just eating less and moving more. Diets are so "yesterday"!

Together, we will work through the 5 simple steps of your weight loss journey. We will go in depth into each step, and I will give you tools and exercises to use and do at home, so that you can get a real feel for each step and how it can be applied to you.

I will be sharing many of my clients' stories to show you how the steps have been used and implemented in different ways, to suit different lifestyles.

We are all different: we all live differently, and have different backgrounds, traditions and commitments. Which means that each step will look different for you than for your friend once implemented in your life.

There is no "one size fits all". Get the basics right, and you will see results.

As you work through the exercises in each part of this book, you will define your own personal plan, and feel empowered to act upon it. The changes you make will have a much bigger impact than just on your weight. Every change you make in one of the steps will have a ripple effect on the other ones. But more importantly it will have a ripple effect on your environment and the people around you.

The way you look at your life and your health will be different. You will feel empowered, in control, and in charge of your health and weight for the rest of your life.

Over the years, major and life-changing events will happen. They will require you to adapt and change to maintain your results. Grab hold of the book again, and work through the exercises and steps again from where you are at that moment in time.

There will be ups, downs and plateaux along the journey. It's part of the process, and something you will learn to embrace. I wish I could tell you there was a magic pill you could take which would make you slim, fit and healthy overnight. Unfortunately, there isn't.

Try to read the book in the order it's been written in.

You have probably heard some of the points made in the book before. What makes it different and powerful is the **combination** of the 5 steps. All 5 steps are interlinked. Work in small chunks on all of them, and you will see big improvements all round.

If you focus only on one of the steps, then as with most traditional diets you will keep on getting stuck. Trust the process. It's one that has worked for my clients over the past 10 years and continues to work.

Do the exercises as you go through the book to prepare your own individualised plan for the slimmer, fitter, healthier, more confident and happier you.

You can download all the exercises here:
https://anneiarchy.com/5-simple-steps-companion-sheets/

I would like to invite you to join my online community on Facebook, where you can ask me any questions related to the book, share your journey, share your a-ha moments, and chat with like-minded people on their own journey. https://www.facebook.com/groups/ItsNotAboutTheScales

Let's do this together!

PART 1
THE PROBLEM

▓ WEIGHT LOSS IN NUMBERS

Numbers are never exciting, but it's important to realise how much of a problem obesity really is today and in the future. In February 2018, the World Health Organisation (WHO) reported that obesity worldwide had nearly tripled since 1975. In 2016, more than 1.9 billion (39%) adults, 18 years and older, were overweight. Of these, over 650 million (13%) were obese. 41 million children under the age of 5 and over 340 million children and adolescents aged 5-19 were overweight or obese.

NHS England reported in May 2019 that 29% of the adult population is classified as obese, an increase of 26% on the number in 2016, while 20% of Year 6 children (age 10-11) are also obese. Those numbers are going up globally. As a result, Type 2 diabetes is on the rise as well.[1]

In the UK, diabetes costs the NHS £10 billion each year. It accounts for about 10% of the NHS budget with 80% of these costs due to complications of the disease. The overall costs of diabetes are set to grow over the next 20 years, when they are projected to account for 17% of the entire NHS budget. Diabetes will also increase the costs of social care due to complications.

---

[1] Source: https://digital.nhs.uk/data-and-information/publications/statistical/statistics-on-obesity-physical-activity-and-diet/statistics-on-obesity-physical-activity-and-diet-england-2019

There are around 3.8 million people in the UK with diabetes. That's over 1 in 20! Of these, 3.2 million have been diagnosed with either Type 1 or Type 2 diabetes. The rest have undiagnosed Type 2 diabetes, which is a dangerous situation to be in.

Each year in the UK, 24,000 people with diabetes die early. Diabetes is the leading cause of blindness in people of working age in the UK. Over 100 amputations are carried out every week on people with diabetes because of complications connected with their condition. Up to 80% of these are preventable. The cost pressures facing the NHS will not go away in a couple of years and expenditure on diabetes is rising.[2]

Type 2 diabetes is fully preventable and reversible if not left too long, through a change in lifestyle and by adopting the 5 steps outlined in this book.

At the same time, the weight loss market is growing each year. In February 2019, the US weight loss market was worth a record $72 billion.[3]

With 1000s of diets and slimming products on the market, all promising fast weight loss, you wonder why the obesity numbers are still on the increase. There is probably a diet for every taste and flavour. Every few years, a couple of diets are at the forefront. Right now, it's the ketogenic diet, intermittent fasting, and even veganism is being branded as a weight loss diet. If you're reading this book right now, there is a large chance that you've tried at least one diet in your life.

---

[2] Source: https://www.diabetes.org.uk/resources-s3/2017-11/diabetes%20uk%20cost%20of%20diabetes%20report.pdf

[3] Source: https://www.businesswire.com/news/home/20190225005455/en/72-Billion-Weight-Loss-Diet-Control-Market

Most of the people that reach out to me for help, especially women, have tried many diets, and often have tried the same diet a few times, because it has "worked" for them in the past. I did too. None of them work long term though.

■ DIETS DON'T WORK – HERE'S WHY

"Eat less, move more" is the typical answer from doctors, most personal trainers, and most diets, when you ask them how to lose weight. This answer is based on the theory that if you want to lose weight, you need to be in a calorie deficit: calories in < calories out.

I 100% agree with the fact that you need to be in a calorie deficit to lose weight. However, if it was as simple as that, those that are on very low-calorie diets, even without moving more, would all lose weight quickly and consistently and keep it off forever, while being healthy, not suffering from diabetes and having a great immune system. But that's not the case for everyone – not even for most people.

So there has to be more to it… But what can it be?

Depending on who you listen to, and what diet or weight loss book you pick up, the reason for being unsuccessful at "eat less" will be something that has to be banned. A specific food group or a specific food is affecting your results and as such must be banned… cutting out the carbohydrates, or going low-fat, or having only plant-based protein, cutting out gluten, wheat, dairy, etc. I'm sure you've heard it and probably tried it all.

The second option for eating less is restricting the timespan for eating, such as intermittent fasting, not eating after a certain time, having to wait before you can eat again, and so on.

The third option is all about replacing real food with shakes, ready meals and pills that are very limited in calories and supposed to give you all the nutrients your body needs to function properly.

There are a few issues with all those ways of eating less, or "diets".

Prescriptive

Of course, it's easy when a person or a book or a programme tells you what you can and can't eat, and you just follow a plan. You don't have to think. You just follow the meal plans day by day. And if the diet includes some exercise, you try to do that as well.

But is that plan really fitting into your life so that you can keep up with it year after year? Can you get hold of all the ingredients? Do you even like the food you're supposed to eat?

Back in my corporate job, one of my colleagues started a new diet. It was super prescriptive to the point where she knew exactly what to eat at each meal and at what time. One day, she walked into the office and was a little bit grumpy. She couldn't find lamb's lettuce which was part of her lunch that day. So she replaced it with some other lettuce, but obviously that meant she had "failed" to follow her diet.

That same week, we were all sitting in a team meeting, and she opened her Tupperware box and started to eat. It was 11 a.m. Whatever she was eating was quite smelly, so we all looked at her in disgust. She told us she had to eat this meal at this particular time, otherwise she would be out of sync with her diet.

To no one's surprise that diet was very short-lived, as it was just way too prescriptive.

Restrictive

Is what you are cutting out of your diet really something you can live without for the rest of your life? Or is it OK for just a few months until you reach your target? What happens after that?

> *Dry January or Stoptober where people give up alcohol for a month are typical examples of this. In January this is to give the liver a bit of respite after the holiday indulgence. And in October it is to prepare the liver for the pre-Christmas outings and the holiday season. Lately, Veganuary (a month of going vegan) has been added to the mix.*

For 99% of those following the programme, the first day after the end of the month is a massive binge day. Everyone on Facebook is talking about the upcoming pub visit, followed by a big, juicy steak. And from there onwards it all goes back to before the restrictions.

Cutting out the carbs is another example, where people moan that they can't have this or that, and how much they long for a nice baguette, only to go for a massive binge once "willpower" runs out.

Complex

Many diets have so many rules that it makes them very complex. As long as you can focus on the complexity, all goes well. But what happens when life becomes a little more hectic and it all becomes too overwhelming?

> *Ash was on a "weigh everything and put into a special app" diet that was calculating every little bit of food and drink he put into his mouth. After every meal, he had to check what he could have for the remainder of the day. It required quite a lot of attention to detail. However, it worked really well for him. He lost weight and felt better. When the company he worked for merged with another one, and his role changed, he started travelling a lot. Weighing his food when he was eating out was just impossible. That meant the end of his diet, and soon he put most of the weight back on.*

Not Adaptable

What happens when you start moving more? Do you keep eating the same? What are you supposed to do when you go on holidays? Or you're invited to a celebration, or just a dinner out?

> *Sarah went on an all-inclusive holiday, which also included 2 drinks a night. The place was lovely, the beach had beautiful white sand, and the water was blue. What should have been a lovely holiday with her family turned out to be one of the worst she's ever been on. Every time she looked at the buffet, she felt like she was letting herself down by picking at things that were not part of her diet. And although she had only 1 of the 2 drinks a day, she felt very, very guilty. She didn't know how to keep up with her diet while on holiday.*

Eating too little

Do you actually know how much you should be eating to function at optimal level? Or are you starving yourself following a specific diet, feeling tired, grumpy, and not able to do all the things you would like to do due to lack of energy and massive cravings?

> *Many of my potential clients come to me telling me that they barely eat, and still don't lose the weight they want to lose. They might have lost a little to start with, but then it all plateaued. That's probably one of the most frustrating things when you're trying to lose weight.*

As you'll understand later in the book, to lose weight you need to eat enough. Find the level that is right for you and allows you to function at your optimal level while still losing weight. It's not just about eating less.

Health

Is the diet actually enhancing your health? Or is it taking away from your optimal health? Does your diet provide you with the required nutrients for your age, phase in life, metabolism, hormonal balance, activity level, and health?

Emma was diagnosed with diabetes. For years, she had been borderline. A loss in the family meant she started comfort eating sweet stuff, especially chocolate. That pushed her over the edge. Her doctor suggested she start taking some Metformin. She wasn't too keen to start taking some medication, but she really struggled to control her blood sugar levels. She then started on Slimming World, and every evening she had her allowed "syns" in chocolate (at Slimming World, "syns" are the foods that are least filling and are higher in calories, like biscuits, sweets and alcohol). After all, as long as it fit into the diet, then all should be well. She didn't lose much weight, and her sugar levels just kept on creeping up. She never got rid of her cravings, and eventually fell off the wagon and stopped trying to diet. The little weight she had lost slowly but surely piled back on and more.

▒ SOCIETY AND MEDIA: PRESSURES AND EXPECTATIONS

There has always been some pressure to look slim, but since the appearance of the internet and social media, the pressure is at an all-time high. In most Western societies, slim is perceived as healthy, attractive, positive and desirable. Anything else is not good, up to the point where being overweight is even perceived as laziness.

I once worked for a company where I was part of the hiring team for a new role.

We saw three candidates. One was quite heavily overweight, and the two others were what I considered normal weight. After the first round of interviews, we cut the candidates down to two. As discussions went on, a few people in the hiring team mentioned that although the heavily overweight candidate seemed to be quite capable of doing the job, they would never hire him, as *"if he's that fat, he must be lazy"*. I was quite shocked and couldn't believe what I had just heard.

Magazines are full of near size zero models, often Photoshopped to portray the "perfect body". The pressure is huge to conform.

We are made to compare ourselves with models and movie stars, however we keep on forgetting that they are getting paid to look good, skinny and attractive. It's part of their job.

Many celebs don't have to juggle family, work pressures and stress, while food shopping, cooking, cleaning, and having a normal day-to-day life. Their job description requires them to eat healthily and spend time exercising. Most have a personal trainer and some even a personal chef.

It's hard to walk into a regular shop and find a pair of jeans when you're a size 12 or 14 and/or curvy. Today, most pairs of jeans seem to be made for skinny legs. A shopping trip can have a huge knock-on effect on your confidence.

The worst in my opinion is the pressure put on mums with new-born babies to lose their baby fat straight after getting the all-clear from their doctor to exercise. As a mum with a new-born, give yourself a break. Yes, eat healthily, as that will give you more energy to take care of your little one. Yes, go for walks pushing the buggy. But don't put pressure on yourself to get back to your pre-baby body too soon. Your body went through a huge number of changes. Your hormones need to rebalance after giving birth. And with broken nights, it's just all too much in one go.

■ FAST WEIGHT LOSS?

When you run out of ink in the middle of printing a document and can have an ink cartridge delivered within a few hours with Amazon Prime, it's incredible and ideal. When you're hungry and the fridge is empty, or you can't be bothered to cook, you can just go online, order something and a whole feast can be delivered straight to your door in less than an hour.

The ability to order anything online definitely makes life easier in many ways. But it has got us used to getting whatever we want as quickly as possible. Weight loss is no exception. We want it now!

Wouldn't it be great if you could wake up tomorrow morning, slim and trim, without too much of an effort? You're probably smiling and nodding your head. You're not alone! You don't just want it fast. You also want huge weekly losses as well.

I used to watch The Biggest Loser *on TV. Obese people, being pushed to their limit, losing 10-15lbs every week. Anything less was a big disappointment. By the end of the series, they were different people. Most of them, if not all, had lost more than half their body weight. They looked and felt amazing. However, once back to their normal life, and job, and out of that competitive mindset and structure, most of them put all the weight back on and more.*

It's OK when you don't have anything else to worry about than weight loss, when you get put through your paces, and get fed (even if you don't like the food per se). But unless you learn how to deal with life, juggling work, family, social activities and a healthy lifestyle, weight loss will not be sustainable long term.

One of my clients, Jolene, said the following:

I have implemented Anne's approach, which is to approach weight loss a different way. I focus on sustainability for forever, making exercise a part of my life – also forever, so it has to be able to really fit into my life. And I am slowly but surely changing habits that don't serve me well. It's been MUCH slower than when I have done any other approach, but I find I don't yo-yo, because if there is a day or weekend I go off track, I just continue as normal the next day. This is not a 30-day cleanse; it's the rest of my life. I have lost 10kg this year so far. I am so chuffed. It may seem little over about 7 months, but my body is accustomed to the weight loss because it is so slow.

It's about accepting that you won't be getting huge losses in one go, and you probably won't even have a loss every week. But as long as you keep going, your end goal will be achieved in a sustainable way. You will get there much faster than by yo-yo dieting and never getting there.

Slow is the new fast. More on that in the Mindset Step.

▓ THE "HOLY" SCALES

It's all about the scales... or is it?

When the focus is on calories in vs calories out, generally the result we expect is a lower number on the scales, ideally every week. It's that number on the scales that will push us to be "good" or "bad" straight after our weigh in, or even worse to give up.

How many times have you hopped on the scales, not got the results you were hoping for, and gone straight to the kitchen to drown your sorrows with a bar of chocolate, a packet of crisps, or a takeaway?

It doesn't get any better going to slimming clubs where a loss is being applauded, while a gain or a plateau makes you feel guilty as you're being asked what you're going to do differently next week, as if you had indulged all week long. Maybe you're even avoiding going to your group from fear of the guilt.

Having a binge or a reward or treat meal depending on what the number on the scales shows is very, very common. The number on the scales doesn't always reflect what you have eaten that day, the day before, and sometimes even the week before. It doesn't reflect the amount of exercise you've done that week. It reflects many other aspects that you're not even considering, and that traditional slimming clubs and diets aren't considering, which we will cover further in this book through the 5 steps.

Thus, acting and reacting with food depending on what the scales show is not the way forward. We'll cover more about how to use the scales in the Habits Step, specifically the Tracking, Review and Accountability chapter.

To summarise:

There are plenty of reasons why the traditional take and view on diets will never help you achieve long-term weight loss.

> You can't control how quickly the scales move.
> You can't control how quickly you lose inches.
> You can't control how quickly you lose your belly fat or your bingo wings.
> You can't control how quickly you see results.

BUT...

You can control what you do day in day out when it comes to your habits, your nutrition, your exercise, your mindset and your sleep and stress.

It's time to look at weight loss in a different way.

It's time to look at weight loss as the by-product of living a healthy lifestyle. A by-product of taking ownership of the process and your environment, taking control of your health, and of what you do, day in day out.

Build your own plan that will lead you to your end goal: weight loss for life. Grab a notebook and write down what comes up for you as you read through this book. Download the exercises, and prepare your own personalised plan. Keep an open mind, and be prepared to try things differently. After all, you have most probably tried more than one diet before and haven't achieved your goal.

So, what have you got to lose? Let's do this.

PART 2
FINDING YOUR "WHY?"

What is your "why?" is one of the questions that no one properly asked me when I was trying to lose weight. But this is the first question you need to ask yourself before you even start your weight loss journey.

You have a certain weight loss goal. It doesn't matter if it's 2lbs or 5st or more. When going on a diet, you would generally just think about your end goal and the amount of weight you want to lose.

The big questions to ask yourself are:
- WHY do you want to lose weight?
- WHY is it so important to you?
- WHY now?
- How is your WHY going to change your life?

This is always something that I discuss with potential clients during our initial consultation. For some, the "why" is obvious. For others not at all.

"Why" do you want to lose weight? And why is that "why" so important to you? "Why" is now the right time? How is your "why" going to change your life?

Without knowing your "why", your weight loss journey is bound to fail. Your journey will require effort, focus, dedication, consistency and persistency. Having a meaningful "why" will help you during those times when you normally would have given up.

Is your "why" related to:
 Confidence
 Health
 Activity
 Example to the next generation
 Vanity

Or a combination of two or more of these factors?

■ CONFIDENCE

Libby is a fantastic graphic designer. On a regular basis, one of the team had to give a presentation about a specific subject related to design. She never put herself forward to present. She felt too self-conscious being in the spotlight.

A few weeks after the start of our programme, she put her hand up to give the next presentation. It wasn't easy, but she pushed herself out of her comfort zone. She felt ready for it, even though she was very nervous. It goes without saying that it was a cracking presentation and that she got lots of praise for it.

Deep down, she had always dreamt of running her own company. A few weeks after that presentation, she asked to drop down to 4 days a week while building her own client base. From there, she took the plunge and went full-time self-employed.

She didn't wait till she was slim to take the plunge. She just needed to learn some of the tools you'll read about in this book and take ownership of her future.

Being confident enough to run her own business was her big "why".

Most people I speak to mention that their weight is holding them back from having the confidence to do certain things in life. Dating, relationships, job hunting, applying for that promotion, getting on stage to sing, play or even perform a comedy act… these are all regular reasons for wanting to lose weight that relate to confidence.

Not believing that you deserve to find a great date because of your weight. Settling for staying single because you're not confident to put yourself out there.

Not feeling confidence in your relationship with your partner, especially when it comes to being intimate.

No matter how capable you are, you might not believe that you will get that new job, or feel you deserve that promotion.

Having all eyes on you on stage is scary at any time. But when your confidence is low, it's a big no-no.

Speaking up and standing out when you don't feel confident due to your weight is very unlikely, and it might be holding you back from progressing in your career or putting yourself forward for any other role.

Could confidence be your "why"?

▧ HEALTH

Bernadette was overweight. Her husband had Type 2 diabetes. He was on the verge of needing insulin injections instead of tablets. He was scared of needles. It was bad enough that he had to go for blood tests every 3 months. He really didn't want to see any additional needles. He needed to change his eating habits and lifestyle, but he didn't want to do any exercise. He agreed to eat the food his wife was going to prepare. So

Bernadette signed up to work with me, and over the 12 weeks she lost 2st. Her husband managed to better control his diabetes and avoided injections.

Health is a big "why" for many of my clients. For some it's prevention when being predisposed to a specific health condition, while for many it's reversal.

Diabetes, pre-diabetes, high blood pressure, under-active thyroid, menopause, PCOS, IBS, anxiety, and recovery after knee and hip replacements are probably the most common ones that I see on a regular basis.

What will happen if you don't do anything about your condition? What does it prevent you from doing now? What will it prevent you from doing in the future, if you don't take action? How does that make you feel? How will it impact your life?

Many people don't take any action when they are presented with the opportunity to take a pill and keep on living their life without making changes. It's much easier to pop a pill. But in most cases, the medication needs to be reviewed to something stronger, and side effects of the medication appear over time, which requires more medication. Although medication is the easy way out in the short-term, in the long-term it isn't.

A few numbers worth noting:

In 2014, almost half of the adult population in England were taking a prescription drug daily. The most common were cholesterol-lowering statins, high blood pressure medication such as ACE inhibitors, and painkillers, including non-steroidal anti-inflammatory drugs (NSAIDs) such as Diclofenac. Non-prescription NSAIDs such as Ibuprofen were not included in the survey.

43% of men and 50% of women reported that they had taken at least one prescribed medicine in the last week, with almost a quarter of men (22%) and women (24%) reporting that they had taken at least three prescribed medicines. This proportion increased with age, with more than half of participants aged 65-74, and more than 70% of those aged 75 and over having taken at least three prescribed medicines. On average, 18.7 prescription medicines were dispensed per head of population in 2013.

The cost of medicines in 2013, including costs for those used in hospitals, was more than £15 billion. More than 1 billion prescription items were dispensed in the community in England – an average of 2.7 million items every day.[4]

Obviously, no one can guarantee a life without illness. Unfortunately, even the healthiest person can contract something during their life and may need some type of medication. But at least that person has taken ownership of their health, and has most probably avoided the most common types of medication prescribed in the research above.

Could health be your "why"?

◼ ACTIVITY

Suzy hated flying. She hated flying not because she was scared of heights, claustrophobic, or worried the plane would crash. She hated flying because of the narrow seats and the uncomfortable seat belt, and when the food arrived she hated the fact that she couldn't properly open her tray and the food kept on sliding backwards.

---

[4] Source: https://www.nhs.uk/news/medication/almost-half-of-all-adults-take-prescription-drugs/
The Health Survey for England 2013. Report was produced by the Health and Social Care Information Centre (HSCIC)

When she was asked the questions: what's the one thing you want to achieve this year and what will you do about it? she just went and did it. She lost over 2st. Within a year, she flew off and really enjoyed the whole experience. From that moment on, flying and going on holidays became a pleasure and not something she was dreading.

Are there things you want to do in life that you can't do because of your weight? Have you always wanted to run, but worry about your knees? Maybe it's climbing Machu Picchu or going to the amusement park with your kids and getting on a ride? What are the activities you would like to do that you're currently avoiding?

Not being able to do something you really would like to do due to your weight is often a good "why" to have. Having that vision of being able to do something you've been wanting to do for a long time is a great motivator.

Could activity be your "why"?

▥ EXAMPLE TO THE NEXT GENERATION

David was 50 years old when he became a father for the second time round. Two major incidents occurred that became his "why" to start on his journey. The first incident happened on a trip abroad when he thought he was going to die trying to climb a not massively high mountain. The second one happened with his daughter.

When she started mimicking the noises he made when he got down to the floor to play with her, it triggered something in him. He wanted to be there for his daughter and wanted to be able to fully enjoy daily life with her. He found his "why".

No one dreams of dying, and many people avoid talking about it. But it's not just about when we're going to die. It's also about how we're going to die, and how we're going to live until then. Our quality of life.

What type of example do you want to be to your children? Maybe you had children a little later in life, and you want to make sure of being there for them as they grow up.

How about being able to play with them as much as possible? Being able to get down to the floor and back up again without struggling. Being able to walk them down the aisle and play with your grandchildren. Making sure you aren't a burden on them as you stay as independent as possible later in life.

Could being an example to the next generation be your "why"?

▨ VANITY

Lisa hated seeing herself in pictures. To the point that on any family holiday, she was the one taking pictures. There were no pictures to be found of the whole family together or of her and the kids. And if one was taken and posted on Facebook, she made sure to untag herself.

One evening, her daughter came home from school, and had to work on a family tree. The tree had to include pictures. She realised that when her grandchildren and those further down the family tree had to do that, there would be no pictures of her with her family at all. It made her sad. And for her, that was the trigger to make a change.

As much as you might dismiss vanity, it's a totally valid reason why some people would want to lose weight. As long as it's an important enough reason for you, it will work.

We all want to look good. That's probably a given. Finding nice-looking clothes and looking good in them when overweight can be a real pain. Even when you find something that fits, you might be shying away from the camera because of the way you look.

Could vanity be your "why"?

Summary:

As mentioned at the beginning of this chapter, your "why" can be a combination of a few reasons described. But no matter what your reason, or what your "why" is, it has to be meaningful to you.

Just saying "I want to lose 10kg because that's what I weighed before the kids" is not a good enough "why".

Ask yourself the following questions:
> What will those 10kg mean to you?
> What will you be able to do when you've lost those 10kg that you can't do today?
> What will happen if you don't lose those 10kg, and potentially put some more on?
> Why is that so important to you?
> Why would you like to avoid this scenario?

Once you get to that first level of "why" and what it means to you, go one level deeper and ask yourself those same questions again about the answers that came up. Keep doing this until you feel something. Until you have an 'aha' moment that makes you realise that it's time to take action.

It's that feeling, that meaning of "why" you're doing it, that will keep you going, keep you focused, or help you to refocus whenever needed.

Your "why" might change over time, so if you feel that you drift away a little, go back and re-do the exercise and find your new "why".

A goal without a "why" is just a wish...

The "Why" Exercise

What is your weight loss goal?

_____

What will it mean to you? (A)

_____

Why is that so important to you? (B)

_____

What will you be able to do once you have lost the weight that you can't do today?

_____

Why is that important to you? (C)

_____

What will happen if you don't lose that weight, and potentially put some more on?

_____

Why would you like to avoid this scenario?

_____

Why is that so important to you? (D)

_____

Then go one step deeper:

Why do you want to achieve (A) and (B)?

_____

Why is that so important to you?

_____

Why do you want to achieve (C)?

_____

Why is that so important to you?

_____

Why do you want to achieve (D)?

_____

Why is that so important to you?

_____

Keep going until you feel something. Until you reach an 'aha' moment.

Once you've filled the page in, put it somewhere visible and read it regularly.

PART 3
THE 5 SIMPLE STEPS

Most diets just focus on food, while some add exercise to the mix. Most diets work, but they only work for a while. They work as long as you have enough willpower to adhere to the strict rules they set out for you. Unfortunately, willpower is finite. And as we all are busy, and living in a hectic world, trying to sort out our weight loss problem using willpower is just impossible.

In this part, I will walk you through a 5-step system that will give you control and ownership of your weight loss journey. Read through the 5 steps, take notes, answer the questions, work through the exercises, and build your own personalised plan that will guarantee long term results.

Referring back to your "why" will help you to define and outline your action plan for each step. If you haven't yet worked on your "why", stop reading, and go back and do the exercise first.

The 5 steps are:

Mindset
Habits and Behaviours
Nutrition and Diet
Exercise and Activity
Sleep and Stress

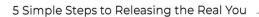

STEP 1
MINDSET

Lack of willpower is one of the most common reasons people quote as to why they struggle to lose weight. Is it yours?

Willpower to keep away from all the food you know you shouldn't be eating.
Willpower to keep off the binge drinking.
Willpower to get up early to go to the gym you don't really enjoy.
Willpower to cook from scratch when you're tired after a long day at work.
Willpower to choose between a healthy dish and something you really fancy when out for dinner.

And the list goes on. We tend to blame it all on a lack of willpower.

If willpower was the solution to it all, why do diets not tell you how to just grow and use willpower to succeed? We all know what we should and shouldn't be eating. So if willpower is what's holding you back, why are you hoping that jumping from one diet to another will change things for you?

We have a finite amount of willpower. Some have a little bit more of it than others. But more importantly, exerting willpower is being in a constant battle against something negative. The things that are keeping you away from the results you want to get. Do you really want to stay in that state of constant fight? Or is it time to reframe your world, so as to minimise the need to use willpower? Reframing your world means working on your mindset and changing your environment. Let's explore how that could work for you.

■ PAST VS FUTURE

When I have a consultation with a new client, I find out what they're struggling with and what their current situation is. I also try to find out whether they've always struggled with their weight, or if a specific event happened that led them to start gaining weight.

For some, their weight issues have always been there since childhood. For most, something happened, such as a big move to another country or town, getting married, starting a new job, or getting pregnant and having small children. For others it's grief in the family, or another stressful event such as caring for elderly parents or for an ill family member. Life events can be a big trigger for losing control of how to lead a healthy lifestyle.

What was your trigger?

Many people blame the trigger and blame themselves for not succeeding at doing anything about it since. It's important to realise that what happened in the past happened. Of course, you could have done this or that, and done things differently. But there is nothing you can do right now to change what led you to where you are now. Blaming yourself for where you are right now is useless, and it won't help you to move forward.

I would even go one step further. When my clients start working with me and I do their first weigh-in and measurements, or they do it themselves if they're on my online programme, I just write things down. Some ask me what the scales said or what their measurements are, and they are sad, horrified or angry at the answers.

It doesn't matter what the first measurements are. What's important is what's going to happen between that moment and the following weeks and years. From that moment onwards, the focus is on the future.

> What are you willing to do right now and every day from now onwards?
> What are you willing to do differently from what you've been doing so far?
> What are you willing to try, even if it's outside of your comfort zone?

We will be exploring all these questions and more throughout the 5 steps.

▓ REAL AND PERCEIVED BARRIERS

Unless this is the first time you're trying to lose weight, there must have been barriers, besides lack of willpower, that led you to stop whatever weight loss effort you tried in the past.

It's important to find out if those barriers are still there.

Fiona started to gain a lot of weight during her second pregnancy. She suffered from post-natal depression, and really struggled with juggling it all, especially once she was back at work. Her weight kept on creeping up. She tried many diets and programmes. But between her work, the kids, and her husband who was travelling for work regularly, her efforts were always short lived. Trying to fit in exercise and cooking from scratch was just impossible on a more long-term basis.

It was important to discuss her hectic life before starting to work together. Why would it be different this time round? She had to think about it, as she was still very busy. But with the kids being older and a bit more self-sufficient (her youngest being 8), as well as her husband being at home more in the evenings and at weekends, she felt that now was a better time for her.

Her eldest daughter enjoyed cooking and was more than ready to prepare some healthy food for everyone. So the barriers she had encountered in the past were not there anymore – at least not as much as before.

For you, though, your past barriers might still be there. And maybe there are new barriers, and potential future barriers that will pop up. It's important to sit down and find a way – a system – to overcome barriers. Review your situation to the full. What are those potential barriers? Are they actually real ones? Or perceived ones?

If they are perceived ones, then it's time to reframe the way you think about your upcoming journey. However, if they are real ones, then you will have to find a workaround so that they don't affect the end result.

Some barriers that often come up when I talk to clients are: lack of time, juggling too much, lack of knowledge, no support at home, too much temptation at work, and a group of friends that are a bad influence.

To be successful in your weight loss journey, it's important to find a solution to your barriers. To build a technique that works for you to overcome your barriers.

Eli wanted to lose weight. He really struggled with snacking on crisps and chocolate. That was always his downfall each time he tried. His barrier! The kids ate crisps and chocolate, especially when their friends came over. He knew that if there wasn't any temptation in the house, he wouldn't eat any of it. At work, he was so busy that he had no time to go and look for unhealthy snacks.

I suggested that he gather the family round the table and explain once and for all to everyone what he was trying to achieve, and that he needed their support to succeed. He asked the kids how they could help so that he would have no access to the snacks at home. There were two flavours of crisps he didn't like at all, and he wouldn't eat white chocolate as he felt it was way too sweet. Everyone agreed that the only snacks in the house from now on would be the ones Eli didn't like.

That was a real help, as it meant that in the evenings Eli wouldn't be snacking in front of the TV anymore.

It's important to be aware of your barriers and to be able to discuss them in a positive and constructive way, as opposed to a negative or moaning way.

Exercise

Make a list of your barriers.
Next to each barrier write down if it is real or perceived.
For each barrier, what can you do to overcome it?

▨ PUTTING YOURSELF FIRST

One of these barriers is our inability or reluctance to put ourselves first. As adults, we generally have our priorities in a specific order and we come last on that priority list, even more so as parents. We struggle to put ourselves first.

Most of us have been brought up learning that we should always be there for others, no matter what. And that being selfish is a bad trait to have. Most of us have been brought up knowing that the most important thing is to perform at school so as to land a good job which will help bring money home to pay the bills.

Yes, those are important. I totally agree with that. But if you can't earn money because you're ill, or even worse, have to have a limb amputated because of diabetes… what happens then? That might sound like an extreme question, and one you might think will never happen to you. Those things only happen to others. Unfortunately, with the stats going up every year, it really might happen to you one day unless you take action. So let's take it a level down and make it more real for you.

Louise's case is similar to the ones I hear from my clients and friends all the time. Everyone and everything else comes first, there is no energy left for healthy eating or exercise, and don't even think of having some "me" time.

Louise was struggling with her weight, but more importantly was struggling with her energy levels. Every winter she was off twice with flu. At work, she was overlooked for promotion on the grounds that she wasn't performing as well as her two colleagues. She agreed she was a bit slower, and as such wasn't always delivering things on time.

Her energy levels from lunchtime onwards were really low. This also caused her to be shouty at home. She just didn't have the energy for her kids being kids, which in turn made the kids even more unruly.

Being so tired she went the easy route for dinners. Pizza, oven chips, jacket potatoes, fish fingers, breaded chicken breasts and toasties were on the menu most days, and at the weekend it was a visit to one of the big three fast food chains to keep the kids happy, before or after their weekend activities.

After the kids went to bed, Louise spent another few hours trying to catch up on work, but by then she was exhausted, so a few cups of coffee and some sweet and salty popcorn kept her going until she dragged herself to bed.

She was way too tired to even think of exercise. She had good intentions to go to her exercise class at weekends, but playing chauffeur to the kids or just wanting to meet friends took the upper hand most weeks.

As Louise struggled with a lack of energy, the first thing we did was to focus on her nutrition. Replacing the processed food and carbohydrate-heavy meals with some healthier food was top priority. It would give her some much-needed nutrients, which in turn would help with her energy levels and focus.

Looking through her schedule, we realised that cooking from scratch every evening was never going to happen. At least, not at the start of her journey. We explored ways to prepare healthy meals in batches, and to use the slow cooker that had been collecting dust at the top of the cupboards. We found recipes that didn't require much prep time and started with those. Once we got that going, we built in a 10-minute workout routine to be done at home together with the kids three times a week. The kids loved it.

After a month, the atmosphere at home had changed. There was more laughing going on. The kids helped a little bit more with the chores and quibbled less. In turn, that helped her to feel less exhausted, and the quality of her work went up, and the time it took her to finish her work after the kids went to bed decreased. She was snacking less, and drinking less coffee late at night.

Her sleep quality improved, which meant she felt more energised the next morning. Focusing on herself and her nutrition, as well as taking those 10 minutes as a family, improved everything. It didn't just help with her weight loss. It had a massive ripple effect.

As her energy levels crept up, she could do more in less time, and she managed to take more time for herself to go for longer workouts, to try new recipes, and she even booked in for her first massage since she had the kids. All that without feeling guilty.

Her boss was impressed with her progress, and when there was another promotion round, she got what she wanted. Finally!

Putting yourself first is not being selfish. It will have a massive ripple effect on everything you do, or currently don't do.

Exercise

How do you need to organise your life to put yourself first?
What needs to change so that you can look after yourself?
What can you start with as a first step?

■ FOCUS ON WHAT YOU CAN HAVE AND DO

Alison started her diet every few months. One of the barriers she felt was that she couldn't eat anything she used to eat as it wasn't allowed if she wanted to lose weight. She really struggled with that one, as she just got bored of basic salads with tuna or egg, or a chicken breast for both lunch and dinner and crudités as snacks in front of the TV.

She got so bored that all she could think of was her usual diet of stodgy food. Porridge for breakfast, or sometimes a muffin when she was out. A sandwich with a packet of crisps and a bar of chocolate for lunch, and then some easy quick dinner of chicken Kiev with carrots and peas and some oven chips. And then nibbles of some sort in front of the TV. Not to forget her biscuit with each cup of tea.

When we think about diets and weight loss, it's often all very negative. We mostly think about all the things we can't eat. After all, being on a diet is being restrictive, right? No potatoes, no carbohydrates, no sandwiches for lunch, no processed food, no sugary foods, no fatty foods...

Have you ever stopped and made a list of all the foods you can have? I bet you'd be surprised at how much is on that list.

I suspect that some foods on that list you have never had or are not even sure how to prepare and cook. But it's not because you have never yet had certain foods that you can't have them.

Of course, if most of your diet right now consists of processed food, it means that most of what you currently eat will have to change. But the amount of foods you can have is huge – it's just different...

Take a piece of paper and a pen, and start writing down all the foods you know you can have. Then go to the supermarket or other food shops, and continue adding things to it. Make a whole list of fresh or frozen vegetables, fruit, pulses, meat, fish, eggs, dairy or dairy alternative products, nuts, seeds, and other plant-based protein sources.

How many more food items are on that list compared to what you normally eat? Can you now see that you have plenty of options? It might mean that you have to try new recipes, dig out some cookbooks, or just look some recipes up. It might mean that you have to learn to try and eat new foods. I know that some of those will taste really nice. There is a whole bunch of foods out there that you can have.

> ❝ *Insanity is doing the same thing over and over again and expecting different results.* ❞
>
> Albert Einstein

Focusing on what you can't have is a sure way to give in and give up. Let's turn it round and focus on what you can have!

■ CONTROL VS CHOICE

My friend Lisa posted the following on Facebook after a big party she went to:

> *I can't believe I got fed all that. And OMG – the amount of drinks that came with it was incredible. It will take me some time to recover from all that indulgence.*

Lisa has tried many different diets since I've known her. Each time, though, the diet ends when she's going out with her friends to one party or another.

It's important to remember that you are in control. No one forces you to eat or drink anything. You make the choice to eat or drink something. Even if the temptation is there, and your friends might be encouraging you to just have one drink or one dessert. After all, one can't hurt. You are still making the choice to eat or drink it. You could make a different choice if you wanted to. You have the choice to tell your friends, family or colleagues that you don't want to be pushed or tempted to have something that doesn't serve you well.

In his book *Willpower Doesn't Work* Benjamin Hardy talks about creating the right environment that will help you to achieve your goal. And if they can't accept, respect and support you for following your dream, are they really true friends? Maybe now is the time to find some other or new friends who will support you and encourage you to achieve the goal you want to achieve. Find some who are willing to commit and take control of their lives just like you.

You make the choice to buy something you know doesn't do you good in the supermarket. You make the choice to skip your workout and not replace it with something else. You make the choice to go to bed late because you're watching something on TV or scrolling through social media.

We have more control than we think we have. And we can choose to act differently. It often has to include a change in environment. If you want a different outcome, you have to make the choice to act differently. You hold the key to your own success.

▓ HABITS VS THE SCALES

The fact that you're in control and have a choice leads us nicely to a scenario I often see happen:

It's weigh-in day. You're anxious about the number you're going to see the minute you step on the scales.

If the scales show you lost weight, you're super happy that your hard work paid off that week. Or you might be relieved that your indulgence from the week doesn't show. You think you got away with it.

If the scales show you gained weight, you're disappointed in yourself because you let yourself down. Perhaps you might be confused, as you have done everything you should be doing, and it's still not happening.

The feelings you experience at that moment – happiness, relief, disappointment or confusion – can lead to one of the following: a massive binge, a "treat" or, as you might call it, a "cheat" meal or day, or a big resolve to try and do better next week.

The scales should never dictate your behaviour, even in a positive way. Your behaviour should always be dictated by the habits you're acquiring.

Those habits that will guarantee that over time the number on the scales will show you exactly what you would like to see.

The scales should have no power over you and what you do. The number on the scales should just be a result of those new habits, and of how well you are managing them. Managing those habits and improving on them is a choice. We are in full control of those.

We'll talk about the habits to reinforce in Step 2 – Habits and Behaviours.

▓ NON-SCALES RESULTS

Another reason why you shouldn't allow the scales to dictate your behaviour is because of all the non-scales results you're going to achieve along your journey.

For most of my clients, the number on the scales doesn't go down quickly enough. However, often I hear comments such as:

> My acid reflux has disappeared.
> I saw this beautiful dress and it fitted.
> I managed to fit into a dress I bought a few years ago, but never got to wear, as I was hoping then to lose weight and it never happened.
> I now walk up the stairs in the office without feeling out of breath.
> I carry boxes around at work instead of asking for help.
> I feel much more balanced when standing in a bus. I don't feel like I'm falling over anymore.
> I tripped, and if in the past I would have fallen over, I managed to straighten up. Felt like in the movies in slow motion.
> People are telling me that I must have lost a lot of weight.
> My skin looks so much better.
> I'm not constipated anymore.
> I sleep so much better.

I have more energy throughout the day.

My blood pressure has come down.

My blood test results are better, and my doctor wants to try and get me off my medication for a few months and then retest.

I went on a first date after many years of being too self-conscious to put myself out there.

I had my performance review at work and spoke up for the first time. My boss was in shock.

And there are plenty more.

All non-scales related results are so important to you and your quality of life. Somehow, we push them back and make them secondary to the number on the scales. But those are the things that are changing your life. So why do you not consider them to be as important, if not more important, than the number on the scales?

And aren't those non-scales related results your actual "why"? It's important to remember your "why". Have you achieved it, even if you haven't achieved that dream number on the scales? Is that number on the scales more important than all the non-scales results?

▧ IT'S A JOURNEY

It would be great if we could all wake up tomorrow living the perfect healthy lifestyle that overnight gets us to our goal. If you're overweight now, it didn't happen overnight. We've been practising the habits that have led us to be the way we are right now for years. Somehow, when we start "being good" and decide to change, we suddenly adopt an all or nothing attitude. We've made the decision, and we expect perfection from Day 1 onwards. Is this really realistic?

It's called a weight loss journey for a reason. There are so many changes that need to happen on that journey. A journey that requires patience, self-belief, self-discovery, overcoming fears, and acquiring a new identity. All that can't happen overnight.

It's going to be a journey with highs and lows. The lows are an integral part of the journey, as they represent an opportunity to learn, adapt, and acquire new skills and habits, while you ask yourself what you could have done differently. We've already talked about the fact that we live in a world where instant gratification has become the norm. Weight loss and instant gratification don't go together.

Your weight will fluctuate throughout, as your body reacts to the changes, and you adapt to them as well. You will have losses, gains and plateaux. Patience is definitely required during your journey.

In Step 2 – Habits and Behaviours, we will discuss daily, weekly and monthly reviews, which are great learning opportunities, as well as times to devise new tweaks and tactics to cope with specific situations. This journey is also the time to acquire a new identity. Who are you right now? And who do you need to become?

■ IDENTITY

Bea was really struggling. She was doing very well with her exercises. But she struggled with her eating habits. "I'm a snacker!" was her typical answer when I asked her about why she struggled so much.

She was leading a hectic life, and she was a perfectionist. She didn't enjoy cooking, but she had someone come in regularly to batch cook some meals. Even with that, she preferred to snack throughout the day and wasn't making the time to sit down and eat. No matter how many times we discussed sitting down for meal times and taking a short break, her answer was that she's always been a snacker. So that's what she was.

That identity was stuck with her for years and years. You might identify as a comfort or emotional eater, a stress eater, being big boned, always having been chubby, having bad genes, never having been sporty, being a fussy eater... and the list goes on. What's your current identity? And how long have you had it for?

If you believe that what you are is fixed and unchangeable, you will always get stuck the moment you experience any form of difficulty or negative feedback. The belief that you can't change leads to a victim mentality. The belief that you can change leads you to take responsibility for your life.

If you've built up habits that lead to a specific identity over the course of 20-30 years, it won't happen overnight. But if you believe you can change and are willing to change, it will happen.

Do you know who you need to become to achieve your goals?

Let me share some of my own identity issues from when I struggled. I always envied those people who looked fit and slim. I defined myself as a Haribo addict (now in remission), but I am still a food lover. I enjoyed sport, but never had the inclination to get to the point where I would spend a lot of time training for it. In my mind, to become slim and fit, I had to eat salads every day and become a gym bunny.

I resisted that perceived identity for many, many years. Every time I ate a few salads, I got myself some cake. Every time I went to the gym, I crossed the road and went to buy some Haribos. Both as a reward for being "good". I couldn't imagine myself turning into a salad eater and a gym bunny. I still can't.

Today, I know that I can achieve my goals without having to eat a salad for breakfast, lunch and dinner, or spend hours in the gym. But that jump from where I was and my identity then, to who I thought I had to become, was way too big, unrealistic and massively scary.

We like to stay in our comfort zone. We like homeostasis. Change is scary. As much as change is an incredible opportunity, it also brings with it some fears.

Exercise

What is your current identity? How do you define yourself?
What's your perception of a slim person?
What identity do you have to take on to become the person you want to be?

■ THE THREE FEARS

For many years, Sue was quite determined to lose weight. Every time she managed to lose some weight, feel better, and look better, her husband took her away on holidays. He's a big lover of food, and loves trying new restaurants, especially when away. A meal out always has to include 3 courses as a minimum – otherwise he feels short-changed.

After every trip, she struggled to get back to her diet, and slowly the weight crept up and up. She had never made the connection between her struggle to lose weight and her husband planning a holiday until I mentioned it.

She had an open discussion with her husband. He was worried. Worried that once she gained confidence in the way she looked and felt, she wouldn't want him anymore. So each time she managed to lose weight, he would sabotage her results by taking her on holidays.

There are 3 types of fears that will come up as you go along. And those fears are obstacles you will have to overcome.

Fear of change
Fear of success
Fear of failure

Fears can be yours, or they may come from people around you resisting you changing or wanting you to fail so that they don't feel like a failure themselves. There can also be fears about the effect that your change will have on your environment. Often fears are subconscious, which makes pinpointing them even harder, let alone counteracting them.

I've mentioned previously that we all like to stay in our comfort zone. You know what it's like being in your current situation. Even if it might not be ideal. It's a safe place. You know how to behave in it. You have your habits, your routines, your actions and reactions. You, and everyone around you, is used to you in your current situation.

Fear of change often holds us back from taking action in the direction we want to go. It causes us to doubt our ability to make the change and makes us wonder how the change will affect us, those around us and our environment. Our fear of change is based on stories we tell ourselves. Some might be real, but most of them are imagined (even if done unconsciously).

Remember the previous chapter when we discussed identity.

What are the habits you know you need to acquire to achieve your results?
How do those habits make you feel?
How will those changes affect your family, your friends, your work colleagues, your family life, your social life, and your work?
How does that make you feel?
Who are you going to become if you are successful?
How does that new identity make you feel?

If you've never been slim, or haven't been for a long time, then not knowing what it will be like can be scary. You're actually wanting and working towards something that you have no clue how it will be and feel – the unknown.

What does success look like?
Are you able to cope with it?
Do you feel you can be the person you want to become?
Or does that look scary right now as the change is too drastic?
Is it the unknown that is holding you back?
Do you deep down believe you deserve to be successful?

Could you break the jump down into smaller stages to reduce the leap into the massive unknown and make it a more realistic journey?
Would that help to reduce the fear of success?
What does success really mean to you?
How is it going to change you, the people around you, and your environment?

If you have tried to lose weight many times in the past, fear of failure plays a massive role in holding you back from achieving the weight loss you want. This fear is also subconsciously self-imposed as we strive for perfection and we worry that if we don't manage it we'll feel like a failure, but also be perceived by others as a failure. It's sometimes easier to not even start than to face the fear of failure (again).

> What would happen if you failed?
> How would that make you feel?

You can't control what others will think of you, and how they will react to the changes you are making to achieve your personal goals. Often, that's a big part of the fear we feel. You don't know if you're going to lose some friends over it, or if your family is going to be fully supportive. The only thing you can control is what you do day in, day out.

Exercise

Make a list of all the fears that come up when you think of your weight loss journey. Next to each fear, write 3 actions you can take to overcome it.

Now answer all the questions in this chapter:

> What are the habits you know you need to acquire to achieve your results?
> How do those habits make you feel?
> How will those changes affect your family, your friends, your work colleagues, your family life, your social life, and your work?
> How does that make you feel?
> Who are you going to become if you are successful?
> How does that new identity make you feel?
> What does success look like?
> Are you able to cope with it?
> Do you feel you can be the person you want to become?

Or does that look scary right now as the change is too drastic?
Is it the unknown that is holding you back?
Do you deep down believe you deserve to be successful?
Could you break the jump down into smaller stages to reduce
the leap into the massive unknown and make it a more
realistic journey?
Would that help to reduce the fear of success?
What does success really mean to you?
How is it going to change you, the people around you, and
your environment?
What would happen if you failed?
How is that going to make you feel?

■ SELF-BELIEF AND SELF-TALK

Those fears generate a lot of self-doubt and negative self-talk.

Do you really believe that you can do it and achieve the results you want? It might just be that deep down you actually don't believe you can. If the task at hand is a massive one, or if you've had many negative experiences, your self-belief will be rock bottom. Unless you believe in yourself, long-term results won't happen.

With lack of self-belief comes self-talk – the way you talk to yourself all day long. No, you're not going crazy… we all do it subconsciously. We talk to ourselves all the time.

I challenge you for the next 24 hours to write down every word you tell yourself throughout the day. Once you've written everything down, re-read all the pages, then re-read again. Would you speak like that to a friend of yours? Is what you're telling yourself really true? That voice in your head needs to be silenced. It needs to be silenced because it's totally negative and unhelpful.

My friend Noelle calls that voice "the idiot on your shoulder". My friend Pete Cohen calls it "the duck quacking away". He even wrote a whole book about it called *Shut the Duck Up*. Whatever you want to call it, it needs to be silenced. A good way to do it is to name that voice. Whenever you hear it opening its mouth, you can just shush it. You start recognising that it is talking to you, and just tell it to be quiet and go away.

Treating that voice as a third party makes the process much easier. Learn to recognise both when the voice starts talking to you and how it tries to sabotage everything you're trying to achieve. The more you recognise it early on, and manage to quieten it, the easier your journey will be, and the more your self-belief will grow.

If you look at babies and toddlers, they have huge levels of self-belief. They are happy to try everything and anything. As parents, family members or teachers we often stop them from many things. At this young age already that voice is being built up. I'm not saying that toddlers need to be allowed to get out of hand, but if you're a parent, be aware of how you speak to your child, so as not to feed their little voice of doubt. Life experiences are already bound to do that.

A good way to overcome that negative self-talk and self-doubt is by breaking down your goal into very small steps. I'm not talking about a weight loss goal. I'm talking about the new healthy habits you're building. Set yourself very small goals every day. Small steps you know you can take. Keep brushing the voice away and, over time, your true voice will grow. The voice of confidence and self-belief.

You won't be perfect at shushing that voice overnight. It takes time and practice. You've been chipping away at your self-belief with your negative self-talk for years.

But by taking small steps, and by recognising when that voice (insert the name you called it) is talking at you, you will feel more positive and grow in confidence that you can really achieve your ultimate goal, not just for a little while, but long term.

■ LEARN ABOUT YOURSELF

I had an interesting discussion with a friend around self-love. She's been struggling with her weight since her student years. She asked me the following question:

Everyone talks about self-love, and I would already have succeeded in losing that weight. But if I don't like myself the way I am, how can I love myself?

If you feel unhappy in your own skin being overweight, I totally get it that talking about self-love is a tricky one. I'm a big believer that self-love will come once you apply self-care and self-respect. Respecting and caring for yourself by treating your body well, feeding it well, exercising regularly, sleeping well and reducing stress on a regular basis will eventually lead to self-love as you see changes happen.

A weight loss journey is an incredible opportunity for self-development and growth.
You might not be a "woo-woo person" – which is what I call people who are totally into mindset and self-development – but since you will be changing, it's a good opportunity to ask yourself some personal questions about your values, especially around self-love, self-care and self-respect.

It's a subject most of us try to avoid, as it can be a painful one. Often our values around self-love, self-care and self-respect reflect aspects of our upbringing, things we've been told, things we've heard, and things we have internalised and linked together.

What is really happening deep down every time you reach out to food that doesn't benefit you? Every time you decide to skip your workout? Every time you stay up late scrolling through social media knowing it will affect you the following day?

Exercise

How do you define and see self-respect?
How do you define and see self-care?
How much do you feel you deserve to achieve your goal?

■ COMFORT AND EMOTIONS

"I can go a whole day without eating and not feel any hunger."

"I am constantly eating – I can't stop. I feel like I have to eat something every half hour."

"When I come home from work after a stressful day, I open a bottle of wine and pour myself a glass. By the end of the evening, I have had a few too many."

"My best friend's mum passed away. She was like a second mum to me. I just couldn't help but eat a bar of chocolate and a large bag of crisps when I heard the news."

"I just don't feel like going out for my planned run. I had an argument at work, and just can't face it."

Are we talking hunger, thirst or emotions?

It's important to understand whether we eat because we're hungry, or whether we eat for other reasons. Sometimes we've trained our body so much not to eat that our metabolism has massively slowed down. We're still functioning and not feeling the hunger, but we're functioning at reduced speed. And no one is ever thirsty for alcohol!

Before you eat something, always ask yourself the question: on a scale of 1-10, how hungry am I really?
If you're a 6-8, it's time to eat.
If you're a 9-10, you left it too late.
If you're anything below 6, you're not hungry and you're eating for other reasons. Worth finding out which ones? Boredom, anxiety, anger and sadness are all feelings that can lead to eating when not hungry.

It takes some practice to stop and ask yourself the question each time, and you probably won't always be perfect at it, but the more you do it, even before your meals, the better you will get at differentiating emotional comfort eating and real hunger.

If you're hungry, eat real food. If not, ask yourself the question: I'm not hungry, so what can I do that is not food related that will relieve the way I feel? Find some displacement activities – activities you can do that don't involve food. Move out of the environment you're in, e.g. get out of the house.

A big question to ask yourself is how comfort or emotional eating makes you feel. Guilty, disgusted with yourself, bloated, annoyed, lethargic and many other negative feelings come up when you give in to comfort and emotions. Whereas, if you managed to stop yourself from giving in to comfort and emotions, you probably will feel proud, contented, accomplished, and other positive feelings. Anchoring those feelings, both positive and negative, will help you for future times when emotions and comfort will try to have the upper hand.

Matt had a stressful day at work. He came home and felt like crashing onto the sofa and eating some chocolate. Instead, he retrieved the feeling of the effect that eating chocolate would have on him. He knew that eating chocolate in the evening was a sure way to have a bad night's sleep. He also retrieved the feeling of freedom and energy a run would give him. He forced himself to change into his running gear and went out for a run. It wasn't his fastest or his longest. When he came home, he felt happy, proud and content, and he got into the kitchen and prepared himself a healthy meal.

Because he had anchored all those feelings and managed to retrieve them, he had the upper hand against his emotional eating and against skipping his exercise session.

Exercise

How does eating comfort food or having that drink really help you?
Is eating that food or drinking that drink really respecting yourself?
How will you feel after eating or drinking it?
What else can you do to help yourself? What displacement activities could you do?
How will you feel if you manage to use one of the displacement activities?

■ COMPARISONITIS

A sure way to struggle on your journey is to compare yourself to others. If in the past you would compare yourself to your immediate circle of friends, family and colleagues, nowadays comparisonitis has been amplified by the existence of social media.

It's important to remember that you are unique. You live your own life, with your own stresses and commitments, and have your own unique metabolism and gut flora. Even if you were eating the same food and doing the exact same exercise as your best friend, your results would be different. Focus on your own journey, one day at a time.

A typical example is those celebrities who lost their baby weight in no time and look amazing at lightning speed. Remember that they get paid to look like that. It's part of their job description. And since it's part of their job, they take the time during their day to exercise, and they eat healthy meals. They make it a priority. Often that happens with the help of a trainer or a personal chef. They make sure they sleep well at night by having a night nurse or au pair who wakes up when their baby cries, so that they can look rested for the day in front of the camera. Does that sound remotely similar to your environment?

There is so much pressure to look like x or z, but we never stop to ask ourselves how our lives are different to theirs.

▧ ASKING FOR HELP

If asking for help and paying for it seems to come naturally to celebrities, it's something that most of us struggle with. Asking for help is something that we aren't good at. Asking for help is often perceived as admitting defeat. Admitting that we aren't superheroes who can sort out our own problems.

We aren't expected to be good at everything. And we definitely aren't expected to be perfect. It's OK to ask for help. It will help you to achieve your results faster and with more ease. Reach out to a professional, and you will get massive support and accountability, which is especially important when you have tricky days.

But remember, the help you receive is not outsourcing your efforts. Your helper, be it a trainer, a chef or a coach, can't do the work for you. If you hire a personal trainer, you still need to show up for your sessions and do the exercise. If you hire a chef to cook you healthy meals, you still need to eat them rather than leaving the prepared meals and eating a bar of chocolate instead. If you hire a coach to work with you on some blocks you feel you encounter, you still need to do the personal work that your coach is setting out for you. No matter how much help you hire, you are the one who still needs to do the work.

Debs got some amazing results. She really changed her eating habits, cut out the processed food and all the chocolate she was eating, and started cooking from scratch. She had started walking more and seeing some good results when she had a fall and broke some bones in different places. She was very disappointed as she finally felt that things had shifted for her.

She knew she needed some help. Especially for showering and cleaning. I suggested that, so as not to break her new habits, she also hired a cook. Which she did. Debs gave the cook some recipes she wanted her to prepare and asked her to batch cook food for the week to come.

For 6 weeks, while she couldn't cook herself, she hired some help. During those 6 weeks, she still managed to lose more weight. Her specialist was very impressed by the speed at which she had healed, and told her that her healthy eating habits had played a big part in it.

Debs could easily have reverted to takeaways and chocolate. But she decided to reach out and ask for help. Being very independent, that wasn't an easy thing to do. But in the end, she was very happy that she did.

How do you currently feel about asking for help? What type of help could make a big difference for you in terms of your weight loss journey? Discuss these with the people around you to get ideas on how to make it a reality.

Remember to join my community of likeminded people in my Facebook group *It's Not About the Scales.*

Summary:

Starting a weight loss journey with a different mindset is key. It's an underlying factor in all the other steps that we're going to work on.

There are lots of questions to work through, and some will feel uncomfortable. But once you work through them, and answer them honestly, everything else will flow much more easily.

And remember, it's a journey. Your life is a busy one, so it will take more time than if you had nothing else going on in your life. Work on yourself and add things in bit by bit as your self-belief grows. That way, you can establish a lifestyle that is sustainable long term.

STEP 2
HABITS AND BEHAVIOURS

Building and ingraining healthy habits that will help you to achieve your goals is a very important aspect of weight loss that is often neglected and ignored.

When I hear people speak about their weight loss efforts, I often hear about the "bad" habits they are trying to break. They get frustrated because each time they try to break their bad habits, it works for a short while, but then those habits pop back up. Eventually taking them back to square one.

In his book *The Power of Habit*, Charles Duhigg mentions that it's nearly impossible to "break" habits. However, to change our habits we should build new and positive habits that benefit us. Repeat them over and over again until the old/bad habits become obsolete.

In this step, I want to cover the new, healthy and beneficial habits you need to work on, repeat and ingrain to build long-lasting results. The first step for each habit we're going to cover is to observe what you're currently doing. Know where you're at right now and build up from there.

■ PLANNING AND PREPARATION

Unless you are retired with no interests at all or living on a deserted island with no growth, animals or belongings, you are probably very busy and time poor.

Planning and preparation will be key to success to combat the "I'm too busy to…" and "I have no time to…" excuses. As we are all different, planning and preparation can take on different forms. It's up to you to decide which form fits in with your life and works well for you.

Growing up, my mum planned our main meals out for the week. Except for Saturdays, we knew exactly what we were going to eat for our main meal every day of the week, week in, week out, and probably even year in, year out. I can still recall the daily menu to this day.

A variety of this method is planning your meals a week in advance while varying the menu from week to week. My friend, Noelle, who runs a very successful personal training business in North Wales, has a blackboard in her kitchen. Her main meals are mapped out every week for the whole week. She also has a master-list of everything they like to eat as a family, which makes the mundane weekly menu planning a doddle.

Personally, and as a reaction to how I grew up, I plan my meals only one day ahead. Every evening I check my diary for the following day, and I decide what I am going to eat the next day for both lunch and dinner based on what I have in the fridge, freezer and larder. I don't include breakfast in my planning, as that's quite easy for me.

My method is not as bulletproof as the previous two methods. I do end up stuck here and there when I forget to defrost some ingredients. So some willpower and creativity are needed if you follow my method.

There is no right or wrong way to plan and prepare your menus. Your method has to work for you and fit nicely into your life and lifestyle. Planning your menus is there to make your life easier when it comes to healthy eating. Unless you have planned and prepared, the chances of eating a healthy meal are massively reduced. Despite good intentions, the chances of you stopping to shop for and prepare a healthy meal are very low when you're tired, hungry or in a rush.

With good planning we're generally covered for breakfast and dinner. But what happens at lunchtime? What do you eat for lunch when at work? Do you bring your food with you, or do you rely on whatever is available wherever you are?

Throughout my career in the corporate world, I mostly relied on buying lunch out. I very rarely brought lunch in. Which probably explains why I struggled with my weight during all those years.

You might have a canteen at work, and some of the food on offer will be healthy, you might go to the local café or restaurant and eat out, you might take food back to the office, or you might go out and grab a sandwich. Or you might just skip lunch and then hit the vending machine mid-afternoon. Which one are you?

There are lots of reasons why bringing your own lunch will help you to achieve your weight loss goals. Many of these reasons will be elaborated on in the Nutrition and Diet step.

When eating out, you don't know how the food has been cooked or what extra ingredients have been added to your food to make it taste good. And it's nearly impossible to control portion sizes. We don't have to eat it all, but once food is on our plates, it's hard to stop eating if there is just that bit left over, even when we feel full.

In no way am I saying don't ever eat out, but if you want to achieve your weight loss goals, and keep the weight off, then leave eating out for special occasions and adopt some of the techniques we will discuss in the Nutrition and Diet step.

Planning and preparation don't stop with food.

If you don't properly plan and diarise your exercise sessions, and don't prepare the necessary clothes and equipment, it's very easy to skip your session. And unless you have specifically prepaid for that session, and the price is significant enough, any excuse that comes up could derail you from making it to your session.

When can you realistically exercise throughout the week? Are you an early morning person? Do you have time at lunchtime? Will you go straight from work? Or after the kids have gone to bed? Be honest with yourself, see what could work best for you, and stick it in the diary.

Personally, I never thought of myself as a morning person. I would get up at silly o'clock to catch a flight or a train or get on the motorway for work meetings. But no way would I get up earlier to exercise.

Still today, you wouldn't see me lift weights early morning. However, since I discovered the benefits to my focus and energy levels after a 7 a.m. swim, I will definitely get up earlier for a swim or potentially a spinning class. Anything that requires some thinking such as a strength training session will not happen early morning.

We'll discuss the benefits of morning vs evening in Step 4 – Exercise and Activity.

Planning and preparing your sleeping routine and environment are also key. And your stress buster activities need to be planned and prepared as well. More on those in Step 5 – Sleep and Stress.

Being realistic, even the best planned days might end up being messed around due to unforeseen circumstances. When we don't stick to our plan, we generally feel like we have somehow failed. When that happens too regularly, we eventually tend to give up.

So here is a great method to always feel like you are sticking to your plan no matter what.

The 3-scenario method

Make a list of all the things you would do during an ideal day. A day where everything goes to plan – we'll call that scenario A. Morning routine, meals taken to work, exercise scheduled and kit ready, regular breaks to move and eat, evening routine, in bed by a specific time, etc. Everything you would do for yourself and your weight loss journey on an ideal day.

From that list, tick all the things you would still do if you were a bit stretched for time – we'll call that scenario B.

Make a third list of the strict minimum you can commit to do every day, no matter what happens during the day – we'll call that scenario C.

When you have an ideal day, stick to scenario A.
When you're stretched for time, stick to scenario B.
When you have one of those crazy days that hit you from nowhere, stick to scenario C.

It's a great way to never feel like you've failed, and to still stick to a plan. You most probably will achieve scenario B on most days, with a few days of scenario A, and a few instances of scenario C. As long as you achieve 95% of the days between A and B, you're doing brilliantly.

Knowing exactly what you want to achieve every day is a great way to set you up for success.

To sum it up:

❝ *A goal without a plan is just a wish.* **❞**

Antoine de Saint-Exupéry

❝ *A weight loss journey without planning and preparation is guaranteed to fail.* **❞**

Anne Iarchy

▪ FOOD SHOPPING

Food shopping is a big part of the preparation and an important habit to acquire. My mum's rigid planning made food shopping super easy and fast. There was no online shopping at the time, but if there had been, then using her planning method and combining it with online shopping, you would just reorder the same shopping list once a week, which would make the whole process fast and easy. Job done!

With Noelle's way of planning, you would know exactly what ingredients to get every week. And since she's in a small village, she can do a weekly online shop and get it all delivered, saving money and reducing impulse buying, while saving a lot of time as well.

I food shop when I have time, I buy in bulk when items are on offer (there goes the "healthy food is expensive" excuse), and if that means separating packs of fresh meat or fish into individual portions and freezing them for later use, then that's what I do.

I love a good farmers' market with all its colours, but I also like to walk the aisles and see what's on offer and buy accordingly. I love to see how marketing works. How new products are being introduced into shops and exposed to buyers, and what they are. You will often see me turn a food item round to read the food label.

Walking the aisles, however, can be very dangerous, especially when you are hungry! The original research by Dr Wansink from 2013[5] has been retracted a few years ago due to his methods and integrity. But his research showed that when people went out food shopping while hungry, they were more likely to buy more than they needed, including some high calorific items they hadn't intended to buy.

From the questionnaire I sent out while doing some research for this book, 90% of respondents replied that they were more likely to buy some unhealthy snacks they didn't intend to buy when going food shopping while hungry. Only 10% were sticking to their list when hungry.

Special offers are another interesting pitfall of food shopping. And from a supermarket and food manufacturer point of view, an incredible way to make more money by making us buy more.

Research by Professor Paul Dobson in 2010 shows that price promotions account for half of all spending on alcohol and soft drinks. Price promotions are also extensively used on ready meals, confectionery, snacks, meat, sauces and yoghurts. Special offers are 20% more likely to be on food items with red traffic light levels of sugar. Multi-buy deals are heavily used to promote soft drinks, dairy, deli and bakery products. Straight discounts are on average more skewed towards unhealthy items, and almost 50% more likely to have red traffic light levels of fat and saturated fat than multi-buy offers. 'Buy one get one free' items are more than twice as likely to have red traffic light levels

---

[5] Tal, A; Wansink, B (24 June 2013). "Fattening fasting: hungry grocery shoppers buy more calories, not more food". JAMA Internal Medicine. 173 (12): 1146–8.

of fat, and over 40% more likely to have red traffic light levels of saturated fat and sugar, than items overall.[6]

I challenge you to observe what you are doing with special offers and to come up with your own tactics to avoid overbuying and eventually overeating.

Here are a few obvious scenarios that I would like you to check out:

In the run-up to Christmas, or any other major holiday, the associated food items, especially the unhealthy ones, appear months in advance these days. Christmas food is put out as early as the end of August, and Easter eggs go onto the shelves straight after Boxing Day. Usually that happens with a little monetary incentive to encourage people to buy them that early.

Unless you buy and then stick them in a locked cupboard, the chances of eating them before the holiday are much higher than if you were to buy the same item a day or two ahead of the holiday. Which eventually means that you will go back to the shop and buy the same product again. Which is exactly what shops want you to do! At the same time, this has major consequences for your waistline.

What do you do when your favourite packet of crisps, popcorn or chocolate is on 'buy one get one free', 'buy 3 for the price of 2', 'buy 1 get one half price', etc? You most probably buy more and eat more. Try to observe what you're doing. You'll be surprised.

Supersized boxes or get 20% extra free also make us eat more, unless we portion the food straight away. Take your packet of popcorn with 20% more or the "grab bag" packet of crisps. Do you stop eating at the "regular" volume? Or do you keep eating because there is just a little bit more in the packet?

---

[6] Source: https://www.researchcatalogue.esrc.ac.uk/grants/RES-000-22-3524/read

When it comes to healthy alternatives that can be frozen raw or after cooking, these special offers can be quite useful. A great way to make healthy food cheaper. But for anything else, it will eventually end up as extra fat stored on you.

■ BATCH COOKING

One of the most useful habits to start forging is batch cooking. Some of my friends call me the queen of batch cooking. Mostly because I can go on and on about the benefits of it. But it really is a life and timesaver on many occasions.

We're all short of time, and we're all looking for shortcuts. Which is why so many of us look for ready meals, takeaways and pre-prepared ingredients such as sauces. Batch cooking is the shortcut for healthy eating.

Batch cooking can also come in very handy when unexpected events happen such as illness, accidents, last-minute visitors, or even for expected events such as a new baby in the family.

On top of the time-saving benefits, some people enjoy cooking from scratch every day, while others don't. I personally enjoy cooking, especially when I have friends over for a meal. However, cooking for one, or cooking when I just have a short break between clients, is not always fun or practical.

There are plenty of recipes that suit batch cooking, portioning and freezing. Using your freezer means you don't have to eat 5 days of the same meal. Once you build up a few different meals, you have a choice of healthy home-cooked "ready meals" at hand. When you download the exercises, you will also get a few recipes. (Go back to the Introduction for the link).

One thing that often held me back in the past was more of a mindset block. It's what I call the "Tupperware stigma". Being that person who comes to work or goes out with their own food container. I don't take one with me when going to visit friends, but definitely when I'm going to work or to conferences and courses instead of buying food out.

A common joke amongst my friends is the fact that I always have some chicken soup in my freezer. Any of my non-vegetarian/vegan friends who are ill know they can always send me a quick message, and a portion of chicken soup will be delivered to their doorstep.

■ EAT SLOWLY

Steve was conditioned from a young age to eat fast. At school, there was always extra food for seconds, but not for everyone. The fast eaters could get seconds.

Nina is the youngest of four. Her older brothers would eat their food, then grab her plate once they were done and eat whatever she hadn't managed to eat yet. She often stayed hungry. So she learned to eat as fast as possible.

Speed of eating plays an important part, both for weight loss and for health purposes. Digestion begins when you stare at your plate and the smell of the food reaches your nostrils. At that moment in time, digestive enzymes are secreted in your mouth through your saliva. Know the term mouth-watering? Well, that water – or saliva – is full of enzymes that help break down and separate the nutrients in your food. Chewing your food allows the saliva and enzymes to mix nicely with your food.

When you just swallow your food at speed without proper chewing, that mixture doesn't happen. In turn, it means that your food won't be broken down properly at the different stages of your digestive system. Not as many nutrients are extracted, or absorbed properly, hence you're at risk of vitamin and mineral depletion. For health reasons alone, it's important to chew your food.

Today, we know that there is a lot of communication going on between the gut and the brain via the nervous system. Unless we feel satisfied and our gut sends a message to our brain to say that we're full, we will continue to eat until we feel full. The communication system has about a 20-minute delay. By then, we've already overeaten.

When you eat fast and finish your plate, you often still feel hungry. That's because the message from your gut to your brain hasn't been sent or received yet. Hence the tendency to overeat. Most people's meals don't even last 20 minutes. Check your timings next time you have your meal. How long does yours last?

Over a period of time, these extra calories/foods consumed on a daily basis will cause weight gain. So how do you slow down, especially if it's a habit you have had from childhood, like the two examples above?

Here are a few techniques you could try:
1. Put your cutlery down between each and every mouthful or bite.
2. Increase your chewing by 10% every week. Focus on it.
3. Increase the length of your mealtimes slowly over time. Start with small increments and build up.
4. If you do eat with others, try to match your eating time to the person who is a little slower than you. Once you match that, move to the next one. Until you match the slowest eater around the table.
5. Never multitask while eating. Eating while doing something else disturbs the communication channel. Stop whatever you're doing for at least 20 minutes and focus on your meal. I bet you'll enjoy your food much more that way anyway.

Slowing down your pace requires practice, awareness and patience. So…
keep at it.

■ KEEPING A FOOD, EXERCISE AND MOOD DIARY

A good habit to get into is keeping a diary. Especially when you're starting
your journey. But even later on I highly recommend you track what you're
doing for a few days on a monthly basis. Unless you track what's going in,
what you're doing, and how things make you feel, you are just 'guestimating'.

A food diary can be kept in many different ways. You can go super
detailed, weighing every ounce of every ingredient, or follow a more
relaxed route of writing down what meals you had in broader terms. The
more complicated you make it, the higher the chances of letting things slip
after a short while due to life taking over.

Unless you are working towards a very precise goal of body composition,
towards a physique competition, or towards an athletic or sporting event,
you're probably fine with the more relaxed route.

A food, exercise and mood diary will give you invaluable information
about what's going on for you.

> *Libby used to eat way too much chocolate. In our initial chat she told me
> that she didn't really know why she reached out to chocolate every day.
> After the first week of filling out her diary, the penny dropped. It wasn't
> so much the fact that she had chocolate bars in her drawer at work, but
> the fact that every time she had a short break while waiting for her next
> instructions at work, out of boredom she opened her drawer and grabbed
> a bar of chocolate. We agreed that, instead of opening her drawer, she
> would get up and go for a 5-10 minute walk. Within a week, her chocolate
> consumption dropped dramatically.*

Libby had never made the connection between her chocolate eating and waiting for new instructions.

Sarah had a regular appointment with the corner shop on her way home from work just after 5 p.m. She really tried to be "good". And every day she was disappointed with herself. Her mindset was fixed that snacking between meals was not allowed. That's what all her previous diets had taught her. So, when she ended up at the corner shop, she got really frustrated.

On the few days here and there that she managed to avoid the corner shop, she came home grumpy and shouted at her kids from the moment she stepped through the door. She wasn't even happy or proud of herself for skipping the corner shop.

Sarah had lunch at 12:30 p.m. and wasn't having dinner till 7 p.m. when everyone was home. She ate a salad at lunchtime as she wanted to be "good". Looking at the time gap between lunch and dinner, and realising that her lunch was relatively small and didn't contain much protein or healthy fat, it wasn't surprising that she was hungry and grumpy by 5 p.m. and couldn't wait till 7 p.m.

When you analyse your food diary, check for the time gaps between meals. Obviously do also check the content of your meals. All very useful information when on a weight loss journey.

Cheryl was often bloated and lethargic after meals, and sometimes even had headaches. To feel better, she "treated" herself to something sweet in the afternoon. We highlighted the meals and foods just before these feelings, and after a couple of weeks we pinpointed it down to a specific salad from one of the chains that was close to her office. She often bought her lunch there, and always made sure to get the healthier options. We're still not sure what ingredient caused the reaction, but after changing her lunch she didn't have that feeling anymore.

Tracking how certain foods and meals make you feel is another benefit of keeping a diary. With modern food not being as natural as it used to be, and many intolerances appearing at a later stage in life, being able to pinpoint the culprit over time, and eliminate it to feel better, is useful.

Exercise

Keep a food diary for the next few weeks and track what, how, when and why you eat.

Week commencing _____

	Monday	Tuesday
Time		
Breakfast		
How hungry was I before eating it? What was I doing just before having it? How did I feel 20 mins after having it?		
Time		
Snack 1		
How hungry was I before eating it? What was I doing just before having it? How did I feel 20 mins after having it?		
Time		
Lunch		
How hungry was I before eating it? What was I doing just before having it? How did I feel 20 mins after having it?		
Time		
Snack 2		
How hungry was I before eating it? What was I doing just before having it? How did I feel 20 mins after having it?		

■ TRACKING, REVIEW AND ACCOUNTABILITY

So how do you know you're on track? The most common way is to hop on the scales and check what they say.

The first thing Gary did every morning straight after going to the toilet was to jump on his scales. On gym days, he took his trainers off, and jumped on the scales there as well. He was obsessed with the scales. When the number went down, he obviously was happy. When he plateaued, he got annoyed as he thought he had done well. When the scales went up, he felt deflated. Some weeks, he kind of knew that was going to happen. But others, when he really tried, he just didn't get it.

When I asked him what he did in all 3 scenarios, he told me the following: When the scales went down, he allowed himself a "treat". Even though, if he's totally honest, on some days he felt like he got away with it having a loss. When the scales plateaued, he ate something for comfort. Just something small to make him feel better. And when the scales went up, he just lost it for the day, and bought some chocolate and a packet of crisps. After all, he had blown it anyway, so he might as well go for it.

Are you addicted to your scales?

Are you hopping on the scales every morning, maybe twice a day?

Or are you more sensible and weigh yourself only once a week?

How do you feel when you see the number on the scales appear?

Are you happy and motivated to keep going no matter what?

Do you feel disappointed with yourself, as you felt you had a good few days or week, and were hoping the number would go down?

What do you do when you see the number on the scales appear?

Are you determined to keep going and keep to your plan?

Do you allow yourself a "treat" because you've done well, or because you've blown it anyway, so you might as well start again tomorrow or, worse, on Monday morning?
Or do you give up? Because it's just not going to happen.

It's important to track progress. But the way you go about it is important as well and should go hand in hand with proper review and accountability questions.

I would highly recommend that you use the following way of tracking:

Every evening
Answer the following questions:
> How was your planning and preparation today?
> How was your nutrition today?
> What did you do exercise-wise?
> How did you feel today?
> What did you struggle with today?
> What else happened today?
> What did you learn today that could help improve what you are currently doing?

Once a week
Hop on the scales if you want to and write down the number on your tracking sheet.
Or skip this part, and continue to focus on your daily check-ins.

Once every 4 weeks
Hop on the scales and write down the number on your tracking sheet. Take a tape measure and measure yourself as a minimum around the waist. To be able to measure around the same spot each time, measure around the belly button. If you want to use other measures, make sure you can measure each month at exactly the same spot for consistency.

Once you start using this method of 'review and self-accountability' daily, tweak, make changes and improve what you are doing, then the scales and measurements every 4 weeks will show a downward trend.

How large your losses will be is unpredictable as they are linked to the many different parts of your own weight loss equation. But that number on the scales will go down, if you focus and take control of your daily habits and behaviours, nutrition, exercise, mindset, sleep and stress, as opposed to having the scales dictate how you're going to behave.

▓ SUPPORT TEAM

Having a support team around you is incredibly important.

> A weight loss journey is not easy.
> Changing your lifestyle isn't easy.

There will be highs and lows along the way. And having a support team to help you through those is highly advisable if you want to be successful.

Danielle has tried to lose weight many times throughout her life. The times when she was most successful were as part of a group. Having supportive people around her on a similar journey has been key to her success. She needs a team!

You might not be able to convince your family members to change, although that would be helpful and recommended, but at least ask them to support you on your journey.

Friends also need to be aware of what you're doing and trying to achieve. We will touch on what to do when in the socialising chapter. Colleagues at work need to be aware of what you're doing to support you at work as well as during work events. Try to be as open as possible about what you're trying to achieve.

Some people will fully support you. However, others who would like to achieve the same, but for whatever reason aren't doing so, might try to sabotage your effort. Be choosy about who you have around you. Until your new habits and mindset have settled, you might want to stay away from negativity around weight loss.

Finding a community of like-minded people on a similar journey as yours can massively help your efforts, as long as it is a positive and supportive community. That's one of the reasons why I started my community group on Facebook called It's Not About the Scales. I wanted to offer people a sense of community. To be around like-minded people. People who care about their health, but who might be struggling to change on their own. It's also a reason why I started my business in the first place. To support people who struggled with the same issues I had.

Summary:

To be successful on your journey, you need to build new, positive and supportive habits. Ignore the scales, focus on those new habits day in, day out, and you will be on your way to success.

STEP 3
NUTRITION AND DIET

I specifically added the word nutrition before the word diet, as the word diet has such bad and negative connotations for most of us. When we hear the word diet, we think restrictions, cutting out, deprivation, hunger, cravings, and add any other negative word you associate with it.

The original meaning of the word diet is the food and drink usually consumed by a person or group. It's only more recently that the other meanings have been added. So, if a diet is the food and drinks usually eaten or drunk by a person, how can we use that word to lose weight, without all the negative associations with the word? How can we still enjoy our food, without thinking about the fact that food makes us put on weight?

What can I eat when "I'm on a diet", without having to resort to rabbit food and eating salads all day long? – a question asked by Michelle.

I wish we could live without the need to eat. It would make life so much easier – said Anna.

Is it really just a question of "eat less", as the so-called winning formula for weight loss "eat less, move more" claims?

Let's find out.

■ CALORIES

Naomi started working with me, and she knew her "diet" wasn't good. She was eating lots of chocolate and crisps every day. I asked her to fill in a food diary for her first week, so as to get a good picture of what she was currently doing. She made an effort that week and tried to cut out all chocolate and crisps. Something she had tried many times before, and always failed at after a few days or a week.

This time, though, she was determined to make it happen. She managed for 5 days, and then reverted back to her chocolate. As we were having a chat, she told me that she was so hungry that she had to have something to keep her going. And the easiest thing to grab was a bar of chocolate or a packet of crisps as those were always available at work.

When someone wants to lose weight, the first thing they do is to cut down on calories. They cut out all the processed food they know isn't benefitting them. Which leads them to eat less, but leaves them very hungry.

The question is how much and what to cut down on. The answer depends on many variables, some relating to your current diet and metabolism, some relating to your level of activity on a day-to-day basis, as well as the extra activities related to exercise.

If you're an athlete, or working towards a body composition competition, then you would get a very different answer to the above question. And being totally upfront, I would be the wrong person to help you with your needs and this book wouldn't be the right one for you.

For anyone else, I would say let's first see what you are currently eating. Make sure you first eat better, not less, and then look at cutting down if need be. What Naomi did is very common. She knew she had to cut down on the chocolate and crisps. However, that chocolate served a purpose.

It gave her the energy she required to get her through the day. She didn't replace it with anything else. She just cut it out. Hence why she got so hungry.

When you cut certain things out, you have to ask yourself the following questions:

What purpose does this item serve?

What do I need to eat that will take me closer to my weight loss goal, and will serve the purpose instead?

In Naomi's case, the chocolate was used for energy. She had to find a healthy alternative that would give her the energy needed.

The answer to the second question is: start eating real food. Start eating proper meals. Fill your body with nutrients to support your daily activity, while still keeping yourself in a calorie deficit so as to lose weight.

Angela used an app to help her define the amount of calories she needed on a daily basis. No matter what she ate, if she stuck to her recommended calorie intake, she was left really hungry, and was very tempted to "cheat" on her app and eat more.

There are plenty of daily calorie calculators out there, from apps to websites to complex formulas. All giving you an estimate of how many calories you require on a daily basis. From experience, most of them give you a very inaccurate and inconsistent answer. Unless you have to answer plenty of questions about your daily life, and you are tracked for a few days to precisely calculate your basic metabolic rate (BMR) and your daily calorie needs, it's all a big guesswork.

If you're determined to focus on calorie tracking, then I would suggest you take whatever number you've been given by your calculator, stick to it for a week or two, and see what happens. If you are hungry all the time, or don't have enough energy to carry you to the end of the day, then up your calorie intake from nutrient-rich sources.

If you feel satisfied and energised, then try to cut down a tiny bit, and tweak until you find the right balance: losing weight without the constant feeling of hunger and cravings. The importance here is to find the right balance for you and your lifestyle. Don't feel you have to stick to a specific number because someone or some app has told you that was the magic number.

That number will change up or down over time as you lose weight, become more active, build more muscle, get older, and a few other parameters. So keep tweaking and adapting depending on the results and feelings you are getting. But always give it a few days up to a week to see how you adapt.

Once you've achieved your weight loss goal, the tweaking is a great way to find out what works for you for maintenance.

NOTE: If you are a sugar addict and you're cutting out the sugars, the first few days, up to the first week, will be hard, and you will suffer from sugar withdrawal symptoms. You might feel the munchies, edgy, sluggish, headachy and more. Those are all sugar withdrawal symptoms and not real hunger. Which is why I suggest you stick with it for a few weeks before adapting. More about sugar later in this step.

Now the big question is: are all calories equal?

> For pure weight loss purposes only – yes.
> For health purposes, cravings, and long-term weight loss purposes – no.

Let's find out how that works.

▓ FOOD GROUPS, MACRONUTRIENTS AND MICRONUTRIENTS

Carbs are bad for you.
Fat is fattening and unhealthy.
Count your macros.

All slogans we hear on a day-to-day basis in the media and on social media.

So, let's start with down-to-earth definitions. A word of warning: this chapter is probably the driest one you will read in the whole book, but don't skip it. It's an important one!

Food groups and macronutrients (macros) are one and the same thing! Carbohydrates, protein and fat make up the different food groups or macronutrients.

Micronutrients are vitamins and minerals.

Depending on what guru you're asking or what diet you're following, you will get a different answer as to how much to eat of everything, what to cut out and what to avoid.

Unless you want to really learn more about nutrition and become passionate about it, I am going to try to keep it simple in this chapter, while still giving you a good understanding.

We need all three macronutrients to be healthy, and we also need as many different micronutrients as possible too.

Carbohydrates are the first source of energy the body uses.

Carbohydrates are the sugars, starches and fibres found in fruits, grains, vegetables and milk products. Yes, you read that right! Sugars... Which is why carbohydrates are such an easily available source of energy for our body.

Carbohydrates are also an important source of fuel for your brain. They help you to think clearly and not feel foggy.

Carbohydrates are divided in 2 groups: simple and complex carbohydrates. The difference between the two types is the chemical structure and how quickly the sugar is absorbed and digested. You guessed it right: the sugars from simple carbohydrates are absorbed much faster than those from complex carbohydrates.

Simple carbohydrates generally lead to spikes in blood sugar levels and to sugar highs, while complex carbohydrates provide more sustained energy, mainly because of the additional starch and fibre you find in them.

Once ingested, carbohydrates break down into smaller units of sugar. The small intestine absorbs these smaller units, which then enter the bloodstream and travel to the liver. The liver converts all these sugars into glucose, which is carried through the bloodstream, accompanied by insulin (secreted by the pancreas), and converted into energy for all our basic body functioning and physical activity.

If the glucose is not immediately needed for energy, the body will store the glucose in the form of glycogen. Once glycogen stores are full, the leftovers are processed and stored as fat in our fat cells.

Complex carbohydrates are often high in fibre and packed with micronutrients (vitamins and minerals), while simple carbohydrates are often referred to as "empty" because they don't contain any fibre or micronutrients.

Fibre is essential to digestion. Fibre comes mainly from plant-based foods such as fruit, vegetables, grains, nuts, and legumes or pulses. Unlike sugars and starches, fibre is not absorbed in the small intestine and is not converted into glucose. Fibre doesn't contribute to calories nor does it help with energy. However, fibre is very important for our general health and digestion.

Fibre can also be divided into 2 sorts, both present in all fibre-rich foods at different levels:

Soluble fibre, which dissolves in water to form a gel type consistency. This type can help lower cholesterol and glucose levels.

Insoluble fibre, which promotes healthy digestion and bowel movements.

A good example for fibre and the effect it has on glucose levels is when you compare eating an orange to drinking orange juice. When you juice a fruit (or a vegetable), you lose the fibre. Juice spikes the blood sugar levels, or glucose levels, much more than eating the fruit as a whole.

Proteins are the building blocks of muscle tissue in the body, and they serve as a secondary source of energy once your carbohydrate reserves (glycogen levels) are empty. However, using protein as an energy source isn't good, as it means breaking down the muscle tissue we so much need.

Proteins are broken down during digestion into smaller parts. Protein is made from building blocks called amino acids. Because we don't store amino acids, our bodies can make them in two different ways: either from scratch, or by modifying others. Nine amino acids, known as the essential amino acids, must come from food.

Sources of protein include both animals and plants: meats, dairy products, fish and eggs, as well as grains, legumes and nuts. Animal-sourced protein contains all essential amino acids, while plant-based protein doesn't.

We'll go into more depth about the implications of that in the Carnivore/Vegetarian/Vegan chapter.

Fats are one of the building blocks for our cells. And fat also provides much-needed energy to our brain. Without fat, we wouldn't survive.

Fats are made of fatty acids. Together, those fatty acids are called lipids. Fats are produced in the liver, and transported around the body via our blood when they attach to protein. Once lipids attach to protein and are going through our blood, we can call them lipoprotein. And you might have heard the terms High Density Lipoprotein (HDL) and Low-Density Lipoprotein (LDL) relating to cholesterol.

The LDL are the bad ones, which we're aiming to lower, and the HDL are the good ones, which we're aiming to bring up. As I've already said, fat is important, but not all fat is the same.

There are 3 types of fats, and most foods contain a mixture of those different types:

Saturated fat – often perceived as the "bad" fat.
>Fatty beef, lamb, pork, poultry with skin, lard, cream, butter, cheese, and other dairy products.

Unsaturated fat, which breaks down into monounsaturated fats and polyunsaturated fats – often perceived as the "good" fat.
>Avocados and avocado oil, olives and olive oil, peanut butter and peanut oil, vegetable oils such as sunflower, corn or canola oils, fatty fish such as salmon and mackerel, nuts and seeds such as almonds, hazelnuts, cashews, sesame seeds, pumpkin seeds, sunflower seeds and more.

Transfat – often perceived as the "evil" fat to avoid at all cost. Fried foods, baked goods such as cakes, pie crusts, biscuits, pizza, crackers, margarines and other spreads.

Even these 3 types break down into smaller types, but we won't get into those in this book.

Here's a surprise for you: you need fat to lose fat! So forget about all the "low" or "light" versions of food. We'll get to that in the Natural vs Processed Foods chapter.

Micronutrients are all our vitamins and minerals. We need a variety of them, and plenty of them, to be healthy.

Unfortunately, today, even the fruit and vegetables we eat don't contain as many micronutrients as they did 70+ years ago. That is mainly due to the quality of the soil they've been growing in, chemicals that are being sprayed on, as well as the way fruit and vegetables are being harvested, stored and transported.

Different colours of food will provide different micronutrients, hence the saying: try to eat like a rainbow. More on that in the Gut Health chapter.

Something that is important to remember is that food items are often a combination of different macronutrients and micronutrients.

Here are a few examples (all based on 100g):

	Broccoli	Fillet Steak	Couscous
Total Fat	0.4 g	18 g	0.2 g
Saturated Fat	0 g	2.8 g	0 g
Polyunsaturated Fat	0 g	9 g	0.1 g
Monounsaturated Fat	0 g	4.4 g	0 g
Cholesterol	0 mg	0 mg	0 mg
Total Carbohydrate	7 g	9 g	23 g
Dietary Fibre	2.6 g	6 g	1.4 g
Sugar	1.7 g	0.8 g	0.1 g
Protein	2.8 g	23 g	3.8 g
Micronutrients	Vitamin A, Vitamin C, Calcium, Iron, Vitamin B6, Magnesium, Potassium, Sodium.	Calcium, Iron, Vitamin B6, Magnesium, Potassium, Sodium.	Iron, Vitamin B6, Magnesium, Potassium, Sodium.

So, when someone says: "I'm cutting out the carbs", and cuts out couscous, they still get some carbohydrates from the steak and the broccoli.

■ MEALS AND SNACKS

I'm skipping breakfast, said Trish. If I eat breakfast, I can't stop eating for the rest of the day. It gives me the munchies. But the one thing I need is my coffee – otherwise I'm totally useless in the morning. Once I've had a few mugs, I'm perfectly fine.

Should we eat 3 large meals a day?
Should we eat 6 smaller meals a day?
Is snacking inbetween meals bad for you?
Is breakfast the most important meal of the day?

There is no 'one size fits all'. It has to fit in with your lifestyle.

I said I didn't like to talk about calories earlier. As long as you nourish your body to sustain your activity, and as long as you eat (and drink) less than you expend, weight loss will happen.

Is eating 4-5 smaller meals for the sake of it better than 3 larger meals? No, definitely not. It's actually good to give your digestive system time to rest between meals so that it can function properly.

However, and this is where lifestyle comes in, if you have a long gap between lunch and dinner your blood sugar levels will drop quite low, and your mood and focus will be affected. If your diet prevents you from snacking, the lack of energy and focus increases the need for a quick boost, which often means grabbing something unhealthy and leaving you feeling like you failed.

When it comes to deciding how many meals and snacks you're going to have, you need to look at:

- Your (day) plans and activity levels that day.
- Expected mealtimes.
- Your energy levels throughout the day (without the aid of caffeine).
- The content of your meals and the proportion of the different macronutrients.

Some days, you will be perfectly fine with 3 meals and no snacks, while others you would be better off with 3 meals and 1 snack, and other days potentially with 4-5 smaller meals. All depending how that specific day is built for you.

This might sound very contradictory to anything and everything you've tried and heard before. But if you're reading this book, it means that you still haven't figured out what works for you long term. So why not try something different and find the right balance for you…

Depending on what you eat at a mealtime, your blood sugar levels will start dropping 4-5 hours after a meal. Signals will be sent to your brain that it's time to eat. Your stomach starts grumbling. Your focus begins to drop. You start thinking of what you're going to eat soon.

If your next meal is not for another few hours, which is often the case around 4-5pm before you leave work, the chances of stopping at the corner shop on your way home, or of opening the sweet cupboard at home are high. And then your self-talk, fight with willpower, guilt and the feeling of failure kick in.

That's why keeping a food diary is so important. It will help you keep track of times, content (food and drink), hunger levels and mood. Add activities on each day, and you have a fantastic tool to help you plan your meal and snack timings better.

■ PORTION SIZES AND PACKAGING

"Everything in moderation..." – a saying you hear all the time, but doesn't quantify and clarify things enough.

David was eating quite healthily in general. He enjoyed cooking, trying new recipes, and at the same time eating lots of healthy foods. There was always enough for seconds, and breakfast was a nice big bowl of porridge.

As we started making some tweaks to his diet, we mostly focused on portion sizes.

Over the years, we have become accustomed to larger portion sizes. There are a few reasons for this:

1. Plate sizes have increased. Yes, if you dig out your grandparents' plates, or walk into an antique show (and antique is not always 100 years or more ago), you will find that the plate sizes were much smaller. Bowls, such as breakfast bowls, didn't really exist. And even over the past 10-20 years they have massively increased in size. No one likes to see a half full/empty plate. Visually, it makes you think you haven't eaten enough to feel full. The eyes and brain play a big part in satiety.

2. We now tend to eat out more and want value for money, so restaurant portions are large to give us that feeling of value. Our eyes have adapted to those, so automatically at home we tend to make larger portions as well. It's the same with portion sizes of takeaways.

3. Food packaging influences our portion sizes. Food manufacturers have teams at hand to research what the right packaging size is to make us eat more, so that we buy more regularly.

As a result of eating larger portion sizes, our weight has gradually gone up.

Let's go back to basics and see what in my opinion a regular portion size is:

Red meat	130g
Poultry and fish	150g
Eggs	2
Yoghurt	125-150g
Cottage cheese and fromage frais	150g
Hard cheese	a small match box size
Milk	200ml
Vegetables	80g cooked
Salad leaves	1 cup
Fruit	80g fresh (not dried)
Pulses	130g (cooked)
Oats	40g
Cereal	30g
Bread	1 slice
Nuts	10-15 nuts

A little exercise for you:
Over the next week, look at all the packages you buy and divide them by the number of portions. Or weigh your food for a week and write down at every meal how many portions of protein, carbohydrate, fat, vegetables and fruit you eat.

You will most probably discover that you eat quite a lot of portions of carbohydrate and fruit. And under-eat when it comes to vegetables. And if you are a meat lover, you probably overeat protein as well, especially in one meal.

Your 4oz fillet steak is fine, but when you go for a 5oz steak let alone a 6oz one, you are already overeating. When you fill your bowl of cereal in the morning with a hearty portion of it, you often get to 60g – you are already overeating, eating 2 days' worth.

However, those 3 broccoli heads are most probably only half a portion. And what about your fruit? We all know fruit is healthy and it's an easy snack.

Here's what Peter said:

> *I think I discovered why I am not losing much weight. I can easily snack on 5 apples, 2 oranges and a couple of bananas. And I have half a grapefruit with breakfast every day. I have always been told that fruit is good for you.*

Yes, fruit is good. It contains lots of micronutrients and fibre. But it also contains lots of fructose, which is sugar. We'll look into sugar later on.

What have you discovered about your eating habits so far?

Now let's look at packaging.

Most packages show total weight. Take whatever weight it says, and divide it by the right portion-sized weight, and you know exactly how many portions you should get out of your pack.

If you buy fresh meat or fish, ask the butcher or fishmonger to chop and package it according to the above weights. If you buy fresh loose fruit and vegetables, weigh them accordingly.

The big problem you will encounter is that food items are packaged in such a way that will get you to eat more than you intended. After all, food manufacturers are there to sell more.

Here's an example: take two salmon fillets that you buy in most supermarkets pre-packed, or the pre-portioned ones at the fish counter.

Danielle loves her fish. She often buys salmon fillets. But each time she eats a salmon-based meal, she feels hungry quite quickly after her meal. She never really feels satisfied.

Here's why that happens. 2-fillet salmon packs contain 230g. Which means that they are just too small for two portions but way too big for one. But as there are 2 fillets in a pack, you automatically think it's for 2 people. If you're just one, it means you would leave ⅔ of the second fillet. And if you're prepping for 2, you will need to buy 2 packs, which would then feed 3 people.

When we look at food labels you will also see that often there is mention of serving size. Those sizes are often similar to those I described earlier, albeit not always. It's about checking the total weight of the package or food item and dividing it up into serving sizes.

Here again, I challenge you this week to look at the total weight of packaged food, then divide it by portions to see if you tend to overeat.

◼ HOW TO BUILD YOUR MEAL

Here's what Annie told me when we started working together:

I start my day with a bowl of porridge or granola. I make my porridge with water, and I add a teaspoon of honey and some berries to it. On top of the granola, I add a splash of skimmed milk.

At lunchtime, I end up buying a sandwich and a piece of fruit. And I'm always tempted by the bar of chocolate or crisps that is part of the meal deal. In the winter, I might add a bowl of soup to that to keep me warm. Or have one of those large jacket potatoes with beans and cheese or tuna mayo. And when I want to be "good", I have one of the salads.

In the evenings, spaghetti Bolognese is one of my favourite meals. Closely followed by chilli con carne. I could eat them every day of the year. A plate full of spaghetti or rice with the sauce topping is a great way to feel full.

I have some nuts and fruit for snacks, although I often end up at the vending machine, or just have the bar of chocolate or crisps I bought with my meal deal.

Annie is not alone. This is a common picture I see with many of my clients. And the description is not much different, meat aside for my vegetarian clients.

By now, you might notice a few things:

1. The day is carbohydrate heavy.
2. There is very little protein over the course of the day.
3. Annie is definitely not eating her 5-a-day of fruit and vegetables, even when she has a salad for lunch (which doesn't happen very often anyway) or her soup.

Here's an easily memorable way to organise your meals:

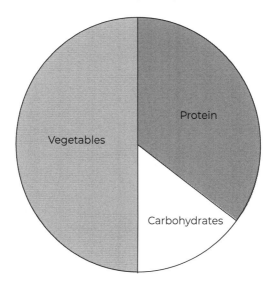

Do your current meals look like this? If you can aim to have lunch and dinner look like this, you will see some big progress in your weight loss.

Breakfast is probably the only time when it might look quite different, as I know you might not be used to eating vegetables for breakfast on a regular basis. If you're not having any vegetables, at least try to have much more protein than you currently have and fewer carbohydrates.

I purposely left the fat off the diagram, as generally you will use some fat to cook your meal in, as an add-on such as olives or avocado, as part of your protein portion, or as a snack such as a handful of nuts. If you have some starchy vegetables, such as butternut squash, swede or the like, then replace your carbohydrate portion with those, while still having other vegetables on half of your plate.

If you have diabetes, you might want to consider replacing the carbohydrates with extra vegetables at most meals.

Let's go back to Annie's meals.

Annie started her day with porridge made with water, a little honey and some berries. All those are carbohydrate and there's no protein at all (oats do contain some protein, but not enough to be counted as a portion of it). I suggested that she cook her porridge with a glass of milk and replace the honey with some cinnamon.

When she had her granola with a splash of milk, I suggested that she swap the granola (which was sugar rich) with some oats, sliced nuts, a teaspoon of mixed seeds, a teaspoon of raisins, and a small pot of natural Greek yoghurt.

Lunchtime was a bit more complex, as it all depended on what was available near to where she works.

However, no matter where you are, there is definitely loads more available than the sandwich meal deal. And there is always the preferred option of bring your own. Even if you buy food, take the structure of veg, protein and carbs into account.

Dinner was actually quite easy to sort out. The big plate of spaghetti or rice obviously doesn't match the new structure. But that doesn't mean that spaghetti or rice is bad per se. It's just the issue of portion size.

If you fill half your plate with vegetables, make sure you have enough protein in the sauce or the chilli, and have a bit of spaghetti or rice with it, then you can have these two options. Or even use chickpea or red lentil pasta to increase the protein portion.

After you get used to eating this way, I would recommend that you consider having a carbohydrate-free meal a day, especially on non-exercise days. Just replace the carbohydrate part with some extra vegetables.

Unless you are in total control of what you're eating at every meal, not every meal will be exactly like the above picture. Eating out, either at restaurants, cafés or at friends' houses can mean the proportions aren't always going to be perfect. On days you know you're eating out, try to adjust the other meals. Potentially even adjust the meals the day before or after.

What's important is that on average you get the right balance – although the more often you get the right balance, the easier it will be to control cravings, hunger, energy levels and quality of sleep, and the faster you will lose weight.

■ FOOD LABELS

After a dinner out with a group of friends, we went back to one of their houses for a cup of tea. A spread of biscuits, cake and chocolate-covered raisins was laid out.

Anthony, who had stopped eating sugar for over 6 months, was intrigued by the food label and amount of sugar in the chocolate-covered raisins. The pack contained 180g of milk chocolate-covered raisins. The traffic light label was all red.

A serving of 45g contained 28.7g of sugar. He remembered me telling him that 4g of sugar is the equivalent of a teaspoon. Hence one serving contained 7 teaspoons of sugar. He was shocked. But he very honestly said that, in the past, he would easily eat a whole pack while watching something on TV without even thinking about it. That's a full 28 teaspoons of sugar!!!

Understanding how to read food labels is mega important when it comes to a weight loss journey. Unless you cook everything from scratch with fresh ingredients, you have to learn how to read them.

A food label generally is divided into 2 parts:
> The ingredients list (with allergens)
> The nutritional value breakdown

The ingredients list is just a list of all the ingredients that are present in the food item. The first ingredient on the list is the most prominent one in the item, while the last one is the smallest part in it. The longer the list, the less natural and more processed the food item is.

A few simple rules to implement:
1. Try to buy items with a maximum of 5 ingredients listed.
2. Avoid items with E numbers and other preservatives.
3. Look out for types of sugar – anything with -ose, syrup, honey or molasses.
4. Avoid chemicals – generally names you can't pronounce.

Allergens – ingredients that can cause severe allergies – will be noted in bold or will be noted separately straight under the ingredients list.

The nutritional value breakdown has to show, by law, the breakdown per 100g or 100ml of product. Sometimes the label will also show a breakdown per serving, but that is at the manufacturer's discretion. If the per serving breakdown is not on there, remember that often a serving size is not 100g. What you eat can often contain more than the breakdown you see.

The current traffic light system in the UK uses the following breakdown:
1. A product high in fat is one with more than 17.5g of fat per 100g.
2. A product low in fat is one with less than 3g of fat per 100g or 1.5g per 100ml.
3. A product high in saturated fat is one with more than 5g per 100g.
4. A product high in sugar is one with more than 22.5g per 100g.
5. A product low in sugar is one with less than 5g per 100g.
6. A product high in salt is one with more than 1.5g per 100g (or 0.6g sodium).
7. A product low in salt is one with less than 0.3g per 100g (or 0.1g sodium).

However, the question of what is better between low fat and high sugar, or high fat and low sugar, makes the traffic light system a little useless and confusing. If you make sure that the ingredients list is as short as possible, you often won't be wondering which option is best. A product can still be high in fat or high in sugar, but there will be less confusion.

Remember I mentioned earlier that 4g of sugar is equivalent to 1 teaspoon? So even products low in sugar can have up to 1 teaspoon of sugar per 100g in them. Note that lactose is a natural sugar occurring in dairy products.

Note also that real natural food doesn't come with food labels. Obviously, that doesn't mean you can eat as much of it as you want (there is no free food when it comes to weight loss and health), but natural foods are definitely the better choices.

Don't be fooled by the design on packaging and by the wording. They are often massively misleading. Full of goodness, part of your 5-a-day, enriched/reinforced with certain vitamins and minerals and many other claims are there to make you believe the product is good, and make you buy it.

A typical example is cereal. To make cornflakes, corn is dried up – dehydrated. In the drying process, all the natural micronutrients that are originally in corn are destroyed. Hence the need to enrich it with vitamins and minerals as per the packaging. It's not extra goodness they add to it. It's to replace the natural goodness that has been destroyed in the manufacturing process and replaced with artificial nutrients.

Food manufacturers want you to buy, and to buy a lot of it. Always read the full food label and make up your own mind. Don't be fooled by bold packaging claims and pictures.

■ NATURAL FOODS VS PROCESSED FOODS

We all know what processed foods are. At least, so we think. Crisps, chocolate, biscuits, ready meals, pizza, fast food, doughnuts, sweets and the like. But there are many more types of food that don't really come to mind as being processed.

"Light", "low fat" or "diet" versions, fortified foods, ready-made sauces, decaf, and – I'm going to push it even further – anything that has more than 2 ingredients is generally processed in one way or another.

Let's talk mayonnaise for a moment. We've all been told that it's massively fattening and we should avoid it as much as possible. However, we all like our tuna-mayo or egg-mayo combination. If you have ever made mayo, you'll know that it doesn't include that many ingredients.

My grandmother used to make the best one. Her recipe included: 1 egg, 1 full bottle of vegetable oil, lemon juice of half a lemon, a teaspoon of mustard, salt and pepper. With all that oil in it, it's no surprise that it's fattening. What's interesting is that her mayo only stayed good for about 1 week – maximum 10 days. A pot of mayo you buy in the supermarket has a long shelf life. Even after being opened! So, what else do they put in it?

As mayo is considered "fattening", some lighter versions came out. Next time you're in the supermarket, have a look at the ingredients list of the different versions. The lighter the mayo, the longer the list. More chemicals are added, and even sugar is added to the mix in many cases. The reason why additional products have to be used is because fat has to be extracted to contain fewer calories. When you extract fat out of a product, it loses its consistency and changes colour. Would you eat a yellowish runny mayo? Me neither… In order to give it a similar texture, taste and colour, additives need to be added.

On the whole, our digestive system copes much better with natural foods than with processed foods. It's easier to break food down and to extract the nutrients. That's what our body has been used to doing over the years. Although your goal is to stay in a calorie deficit, it should be done with as many natural foods as possible to get as many nutrients as possible and stay healthy.

You might be eating fewer calories with your lighter mayo, but at the same time you are giving your digestive system a harder time and preventing it from absorbing much-needed nutrients. A deficiency in nutrients will eventually lead to illnesses, but in the short term can lead to cravings, lack of energy, lack of focus and more. Which in turn makes you want to snack on unhealthy foods. A vicious circle.

There have always been allergies to certain foods. Lactose, nuts and gluten (coeliac disease) are the most common ones. However, intolerances – a milder version of allergy where eating the food item makes you uncomfortable in one way or another without making you fully ill – have become much more prominent as food has become more and more processed and includes more preservatives and chemicals. Another reason to focus on natural foods.

If you are gluten or lactose intolerant or even diabetic, do avoid the "free from" foods you find in the supermarkets. These foods are massively processed. If you look at the ingredients list, you will find a long list of ingredients, with lots of additives to make the food look and taste similar to the original version.

◼ SUGAR AND SWEETENER

Everyone likes sugar. From the time we're born, we are somehow programmed to like it. Sugar soothes us, and somehow numbs pain.

Natural sugar is in many foods. Additional sugar is in plenty of food, even foods you wouldn't think of such as burger buns, soups, savoury pies, sauces, healthy-looking salads, tomato-based foods, and many other products. You will even find added sugar in many food items that already contain sugar naturally.

Sugar comes in many forms: sucrose, glucose, fructose, galactose, lactose, anything else ending with -ose, agave syrup, corn syrup, honey, molasses, golden syrup, inverted syrup, high fructose corn syrup, cane sugar, beet sugar, etc.

If you start reading food labels consistently, you will even see that many food items have more than one sort of sugar in them. This is a known trick to disguise the total amount of sugar in the product, as it allows for the different sugar types to be in different places along the ingredients list. However, if you added them all together, sugar would be far up the list. Which is where looking at the nutritional breakdown comes in. Clever!

Honey is better than sugar, right? And agave syrup is even better! When I want something sweet, I eat some dried fruit, or I have a glass of orange juice. Fruit is good for you.

I often get that from my clients. Their face drops when I break the news that all sugars are exactly the same, with the exception that good quality honey has some health benefits which other sugar doesn't have. Dried fruit is concentrated sugar. And a glass of orange juice has no nutrients in it, unless they've been artificially added. If you've never made your own freshly squeezed orange juice, go on – get an orange and squeeze it. See how many oranges you need to fill a glass. You wouldn't eat 5-6 oranges in one go, right?

So how come sugar is so bad for us?

When you ingest sugar or food that converts into sugar such as carbohydrates, the pancreas is triggered to release the hormone insulin. Insulin's role is to keep our blood sugar levels within a healthy range. The more sugar, simple carbohydrates or processed food you eat, the more insulin needs to be released to keep that healthy balance. When too much sugar is consumed over time, keeping that healthy balance becomes tricky and you become insulin resistant, blood sugar levels rise, and eventually you become diabetic.

One of insulin's jobs is to sort out fat storage. The more insulin we release, the more fat will be stored. Which is why it's so important to reduce our sugar intake to a minimum, and only have it sporadically.

How do you do that when you have a sweet tooth? I hear you! As a Haribo addict, I was wondering the same thing. I tried many times to avoid the sweets but still have biscuits and cakes, or even to go cold turkey, and I failed many times. Often, I just replaced the sugar with some dried fruit, which eventually led me to get back to sugar without thinking about it. The cravings never went away. And each time, I hated myself for falling back into the "bad Haribo habits".

It was only at the end of April 2019 that I finally cracked it. Yes, it's quite recent! That's me being totally honest with you here. I went cold turkey again. But this time I was better prepared. The sweets and sugar were serving a purpose. They were giving me energy, albeit temporarily, as well as giving me comfort of some sort. Although I have always been a healthy eater, I made sure to focus on more variety when it comes to vegetables, to reduce some of my fruit intake, and to further reduce my carbohydrate intake. I am still eating carbohydrates, but much fewer than before. Being more prepared, organised and getting even more nutrients in definitely helped. Another thing I did, which we'll cover later, was to make sure I got more sleep and got rid of my phone from my bedside.

I went cold turkey for a full 3 months. The first few days were awful. I was tired, irritable, unfocused, and just not myself. But once the first 5 days were over, I had way more energy and focus than I ever had with a sugar injection from the Haribos. Especially as it was sustained energy and not ups and downs. I woke up more rested and with more energy as well. A massive game changer was that I didn't feel "hangry" anymore. That feeling of being super irritable when you start being hungry, and needing food right now, totally disappeared. Now, if I need to wait an extra hour before my next meal, I might start feeling the hunger and be a little less focused, but I don't get irritable anymore.

When I started my sugar-free journey, I decided that after the first 3 months I would allow myself to have a dessert on special occasions, but I would stay far away from the Haribos. I have to admit I'm not sure if having a few Haribos would trigger me down the sugar slope again, hence that's the one thing I will continue to avoid.

My taste buds have changed massively. Certain cakes I used to enjoy taste way too sweet now. On the few occasions I decided to have something sweet, I often didn't have more than just a spoonful for the taste. And on my trip to France in the summer, when I purposely decided to have a really fabulous cake in the best patisserie in town, I had a massive sugar rush and felt unwell.

Taste buds do change… So don't hang on to your label of a sugar addict, a chocolate addict, or having a sweet tooth. Not everyone is happy to go cold turkey. But I do believe that it's much easier, as it's much more clear-cut. And when you are then over the cravings, it's much easier to reintroduce sugar on the odd or special occasion without worrying. If you decide to cut down as opposed to cut out, find out where your sugar intake comes from, and cut down gradually.

I was leading a group over 8 weeks back in 2012. The ladies in the group decided to start drinking their tea and coffee without sugar. Initially, they found it disgusting. But they persevered over the course of a week. Their taste buds changed, and they got used to the new flavour. A few weeks in, one of the ladies in the group had a tea made at one of her friends' houses the way she used to have it. She realised how sweet it tasted, and it only had one teaspoon of sugar in it.

Trust the process – it only takes a few days up to a week to adapt.

What about artificial sweetener? After all, that doesn't contain calories or is very low in calories.

The first problem with sweetener is that it doesn't help you to change your taste buds, and as a result your sweet cravings will still be there, even without the calories. Which means that when a regular biscuit is on the table, you will still reach out for it when you crave something sweet.

The second problem is that when you ingest something sweet, a signal is given by the brain to the pancreas that sugar is coming in, hence the process of insulin release is initiated. That insulin eventually has nothing to do to control your blood sugar levels, as they don't rise. Which then just triggers fat storage. The brain doesn't differentiate whether it's real sugar or artificial sugar. It just tastes sweet!

The third problem with sweeteners is that all research coming out over the past few years shows that they alter our gut bacteria for the worse. More about gut health later, but an unhealthy gut flora is not conducive to weight loss.

■ CARNIVORE/VEGETARIAN/VEGAN

I'm often asked what type of diet is healthier and better for weight loss. If you look at all the diets out there, you will see that there are diets for each eating preference. Each one claims to be the healthiest and best one for weight loss. And over the last year or so, plant-based diet promoters have been making us believe that animal sources are unhealthy.

Personally, I don't think that there is a better or worse diet. Some people will thrive on a plant-based diet, while others won't. If your beliefs, religious or environmental, take you in one or the other direction, the only thing I would like to point out is that it is important to make sure that you have a balanced diet with enough protein, enough variety, enough healthy fats, and enough vitamins and minerals.

Being vegetarian and especially vegan requires much more focus and dedication to get all your essential fatty acids by eating enough plant-based proteins and a variety of them. As a meat eater, it's definitely easier to get all the essential fats just from a piece of meat. It's not as easy for a vegetarian or vegan. Remember earlier on I mentioned that meat-based protein contains all fatty acids, while plant-based protein doesn't? Variety and quantity will be key to being well nourished for vegetarians and vegans.

Vegans will also need to supplement their food with a good quality Vitamin B12 supplement which they can't get from their food intake, as Vitamin B12 can only be found in animal sources and can't be produced by the body. At least, not the sort of B12 that is useful for us.

▓ SUPPLEMENTS

Talking about supplements, is it not enough to just pop a few supplements and not worry about eating the perfect diet? Supplements are exactly what the name says: a supplement. In no way can supplements replace a healthy diet.

However, even our natural food, organic or not, doesn't contain the same nutrients as it did last century. Soil quality, pesticides (even organic ones), methods of harvesting, storage, transport, cooking etc all reduce the nutrients in our natural food.

Hence, it's important today to take at least a few supplements as follows:

1. Multivitamin
2. Vitamin D
3. Omega 3 (if you are on blood thinners, do not take this without consulting your GP)
4. Probiotics
5. Magnesium
6. Digestive enzymes (if you're 40+)

NOTE: If you are taking prescribed medication, always consult with your GP before taking any supplements.

Not all supplements are equal, and if you compare the price of supplements in a supermarket with those in health stores, you will see a big difference in price. I would highly recommend that you take food state and wholefood supplements as opposed to artificially made ones. In the same way as natural versus processed food, they are easier to absorb. Good quality supplements will also contain the more potent part of a plant or food, which might be totally lacking in lesser quality ones. Often this will be reflected in the price of the supplement.

■ GUT HEALTH

Gut health is a hot topic when it comes to health, but also to weight loss.

A few years ago, new research came out by Prof Eran Segal and Dr Eran Elinav[7] that our gut bacteria, and our microbiome, define how we react to food, and how easy or difficult it is to lose or gain weight. Straight after it became headline news, a few of my clients decided that the reason why

---

[7] Source: https://wis-wander.weizmann.ac.il/life-sciences/gut-microbes-contribute-recurrent-%E2%80%9Cyo-yo%E2%80%9D-obesity

they didn't lose weight must be related to their gut bacteria ;-) Since then, a lot more research has been done to see if we can change our gut bacteria. And the answer is yes!

Our gut contains between 30 and 400 trillion bacteria. Eating certain foods, taking certain medication, living in different countries, and our stress levels all affect our gut bacteria for the better or the worse. We all know that antibiotics kill off the bad bugs that cause our illness. Unfortunately, together with killing off the bad boys (or girls), they also kill off the good ones. And the effect can last a good few months up to a few years, and even more so if you've taken antibiotics in the first 3 years of your life.

Eating processed food and sugar will also affect our gut health for the worse. Modern research now links the gut more and more to our immune system and to a healthy digestive system. A healthy gut with a variety of good bacteria keeps us healthy.

Eating a diverse diet of vegetables of different colours will help achieve that. Some vegetables that are considered as pre- and probiotics and good for our gut are garlic, onions, broccoli, cauliflower, Jerusalem artichoke, artichoke, leek and chicory root or even endives, and even the Brussels sprouts which are loved or hated by many. How often do you eat those? Do you eat some of them daily?

Having a healthy digestive system means that we can break down the food we eat properly and absorb all the nutrients we need to keep us healthy, energised and keep our hormones balanced.

As you're keeping your food diary, I want you to look at how many different non- processed food types, especially plant-based, you eat on a weekly basis. If you're like most of us, you might get to 5-6 different ones a week. It's time to try to up that every week to 10 or more.

In his book *The Stress Solution*, Dr Rangan Chatterjee suggests that we "eat the alphabet": eating at least one plant-based food starting with every letter of the alphabet every month to improve gut health.

I also want you to look at how many types of unprocessed foods you eat compared to processed foods, and in this instance, I mean anything you don't make from scratch. Try over time to reduce the amount of processed foods, and to increase the amount of unprocessed foods.

Making those two changes will help in having a healthy gut, which in turn will help with your weight loss.

◾ HORMONES

There are several hormones that affect our weight, appetite or fat storage.

We've already mentioned **insulin**, which is produced in the pancreas and is secreted especially at mealtimes. It allows our cells to take in blood sugar for energy or for storage depending on your activity level at that moment in time. Insulin is the main fat storage hormone in the body. To prevent insulin sensitivity, we should avoid or minimise sugar, reduce our carbohydrates intake, eat more protein, include healthy fats, exercise regularly, and reduce caffeine intake.

Leptin and Ghrelin are two hormones that define your satiety or hunger respectively. They're both signalling hormones that tell your brain if you're satisfied or hungry. Leptin tells your brain that you've eaten enough, and that there is no need for more, which helps to prevent overeating. Ghrelin sends a message from your stomach to the brain that it's hungry and that it's time to eat.

Normally Ghrelin levels are at the highest before eating and lowest about an hour after you've had a meal. In overweight people, the signalling system doesn't work very well. Messages aren't passed on properly to the brain. Which in turn makes people overeat.

Sugar and sleep are the two main influencers on Leptin and Ghrelin. Sugar intake, because of its inflammatory effects, and lack of sleep cause a decrease in Leptin and an increase in Ghrelin. Producing more Ghrelin and not enough Leptin means you'll feel hungrier as well as less satisfied. Double whammy!

Cortisol is also known as the stress hormone, because it's released when your body senses stress. It's produced by the adrenal glands. We do need cortisol to survive. However, when our stress levels are elevated over a period of time, it can lead to overeating and weight gain.

Two stressors that are often ignored by dieters are strict diets and too much exercise. Yes, going on an extreme diet and exercising too much is causing stress to the body and raises cortisol levels. Over time, it has the opposite effect of what we're trying to achieve, e.g. weight loss.

We'll look at more ways to reduce our stress levels later on in the sleep and stress step.

For the women amongst us, **oestrogen** is another hormone that can lead to weight gain. Oestrogen is produced by the ovaries and is the most important female sex hormone. It's involved in regulating the female reproductive system. Both very high and very low levels of oestrogen can lead to weight gain.

To maintain fertility during the reproductive years, oestrogen starts promoting fat storage at puberty. During the menopause, when oestrogen levels drop because the ovaries stop producing it, the site for fat storage shifts from the hips and thighs to visceral fat in the abdomen.

As oestrogen levels change, we have to adapt our eating habits and lifestyle. Many women going through the menopause are frustrated with their weight creeping up. It's due to hormonal changes and to becoming more insulin sensitive. Which means that as you go through the menopause, you have to reduce your sugar and carbohydrate intake, and up your vegetables and healthy fat intake.

Thyroxine is another hormone that affects our weight. It's produced in the thyroid, which is a gland in your neck. Your thyroid gland might be producing too much or too little thyroxine.

Having an under-active thyroid (hypothyroidism) means that your thyroid doesn't produce enough of the thyroxine and triiodothyronine hormones. It affects your metabolism, and you will feel tired, gain weight, and potentially even feel depressed. Having an over-active thyroid (hyperthyroidism) means that your thyroid produces too much of these hormones and your metabolism is much faster.

Most people struggling with an under-active thyroid find weight loss a struggle as their metabolism is much slower than a non-affected person's. If this is the case for you, your doctor might be prescribing you some medication. From a nutritional point of view, you can help yourself by reducing your intake of gluten, processed food, soy-based food, caffeine, alcohol and sweet potatoes, as well as only eating cruciferous vegetables if cooked (cabbage, broccoli, kale, cauliflower, Brussels sprouts, etc.).

You can also help yourself by increasing the following:
>Iodine rich foods – seaweed, fish, dairy and eggs
>Selenium rich foods – Brazil nuts, tuna, sardines, eggs, legumes and pulses
>Zinc rich foods – oysters and other shellfish, beef and chicken

As you can see, a healthy diet and lifestyle can have powerful effects on your hormones. Which in turn will all help on your weight loss journey.

▓ HYDRATION

Should we really drink 8 glasses of water a day? Small glasses? Large glasses?

If you search online, you will find a few formulas for how much water you should be drinking. However, it also very much depends on your level of activity, the climate you live in, and even the amount of air-conditioning or central heating that is on.

It is a fact that most of us are dehydrated because we don't drink enough liquid.

Our body is made up of approximately 70% water. Through activity, movement, breathing, sweat, sleep and more, we lose between 1 and 2 litres of water per day.

If we don't replenish what we lose we will feel tired, unfocused, might have headaches, our digestive system won't be working properly, we might feel constipated, have muscle cramps, have dry skin and just not function at our optimal level... all symptoms that we don't always immediately pinpoint to dehydration.

Julie told me that she was drinking loads. The first food diary she submitted showed indeed that she was drinking loads: a glass of orange juice first thing in the morning, 5 cups of coffee, another 7 of regular tea with a dash of milk, and 2 diet cokes. She also had a few glasses of wine at the weekend, which she knew very well don't count as hydration. Even with the amount of coffee and tea a day, she felt sluggish and had that afternoon slump.

We discussed swapping half of her coffees and teas with water to start with for the following two weeks. She was worried that she'd be even more tired from midday onwards, which is what happened on the first few days. But after the first week, she started to feel more awake and have more energy through the day. The only drawback was that she was running to the toilet much more, which was quite disruptive.

We then discussed cutting her coffee and tea down to one cup of each and replacing all other drinks with water or herbal tea. Very quickly she saw some incredible changes to her energy levels, focus and skin tone. She also felt less bloated. And after a month, she stopped running so often to the toilet as her body managed to retain most of the liquid she drank.

Julie did miss some flavour, and the fizz of the diet coke. A great way to get those is to have a few glasses of sparkling water throughout the day, and for the rest, make your own infused flavoured water. Some great options are a few slices of citrus fruit – lemon, lime, orange – some cucumber slices, a few blueberries, chopped strawberries, herbs such as fresh mint, etc. Infuse any of those for a few hours and you have nice natural flavoured water. If you like flavoured water, I would highly suggest you buy a water bottle with an infuser. Another option for flavoured drinks is naturally caffeine free teas or herbal teas. These can be a great replacement for your coffee and tea.

Often, I find that my clients like drinking something warm, and enjoy the process of holding a mug and warming their hands with it. It's not really always about the coffee or the tea per se. Herbal tea is a great replacement for that hand-warming feeling.

Once you're used to drinking more, you will automatically crave it, and feel dehydrated when you don't. Initially, it might be helpful to set an alarm on your phone for every 2 hours to remind you to drink something. There are also apps that do just that.

I have an app on my phone that rings every 2 hours. My friends and family know it by now. When my nieces hear the ringtone, they shout out "drinking time" and we all reach out to a glass of water or a cup of herbal tea for a few sips.

■ FAMILY LIFE

> *Nita was wondering how she would manage to change her eating habits when her husband and kids were eating "as normal". She was also worried about being tempted to cheat on her diet, because she had got used to finishing her kids' food if they left some on their plates.*

This might sound harsh and extreme, but there is no reason why the whole family shouldn't swap to healthy eating. In the same way that you don't need sugar, crisps, biscuits, chocolate and cake as part of your diet, your kids and partner don't either. The reason you are struggling with your weight today is because, over the years, you have indulged in foods that didn't benefit your health. So why would you want your family to struggle with that as well?

Involve the whole family in a lifestyle change. They might moan initially, but soon enough it will be part of the norm at home. Your children are looking up at you, so be the example.

If you aren't a parent but a prominent person in young peoples' lives, remember that you are a role model to the next generation. Whatever you do or don't do, your attitude towards a healthy lifestyle has an influence on them and a ripple effect.

> *Gill has been struggling with her diet since childhood. Her mum had a love-hate relationship with food. She was always on a diet, but at the same time binged on unhealthy foods. As punishment for her mum's struggle, Gill has been put on diet after diet. Her unhealthy relationship with food*

stems from there. And today, it's a tough one to break. She made a real effort not to pass that onto her own children.

Very few kids are fussy eaters from birth. Often, they become fussy eaters when they start eating too much of the processed food that is prepared in such a way that hooks them. Fish fingers, chicken nuggets, oven chips and ketchup have been highly crafted combining the right proportions of salt, sugar and fat, which are not present in home-cooked natural foods. Even earlier, all the pre-prepared toddlers' food pots and pouches are made with ingredients that help develop a sweet palate.

Sometimes, big changes such as starting school trigger a change in eating habits in children. It's worth being aware of it to help them keep on the right track. But as a rule, get the whole family on board. It will make things much easier for you, and they will thank you at some point later on in their lives.

■ SOCIAL LIFE

Before I set up my online programme, Slimmer U Club, I had a call from Emily. She wanted to lose some weight and knew she had to do something. During our chat, I explained that my programmes were 12 weeks long as a minimum. She told me she could only start a few months later because she had so many social events coming up. And then she remembered that she actually had a wedding to attend 5 months later and was going away for it. It wasn't really realistic to start a 12-week programme as she couldn't commit to being "good" for 12 weeks.

Social life is a big part of our lives. We eat out more, we see friends more – even if it's not for a whole dinner, but just for coffee or a drink. There are more parties to attend. It's just part of life, and that won't change. It's important to learn how to deal with those moments when it comes to your nutrition.

Eating out or entertaining generally provides more temptation, and when out you have little or no control of what's been put on the table, and how it is cooked. There are a few scenarios that need covering: entertaining, eating out at friends' houses, eating out in restaurants, birthdays, weddings and special occasions, coffee out, and after-work drinks.

When you entertain, you generally want to make a good impression. For many, food is a way to say "I love you" and to show respect for others. That usually comes with having food in abundance, as well as making sure it all looks and tastes nice.

When entertaining, you are in full control of what goes on the table and on your plate. Again, as with family life, eating healthy food can easily be extended to your friends as well. Healthy eating as we've seen just means good quality protein, colourful vegetables and some carbohydrate. Putting a beautiful-looking colourful fruit platter on the table for dessert generally has a bigger wow factor in my house than having a few regular-looking cakes. It's easy to prepare a 3-course healthy menu that will be well received by your guests. Of course, it takes more time to prepare than sticking a frozen pizza in the oven. But if you are already cooking, there is no difference in cooking a healthy or an unhealthy meal.

Eating out at friends' houses can be trickier. Something that is now much more common with friends is to ask if there is anything you can bring along to alleviate the burden on the host. Instead of waiting for the bottle of wine answer, why not suggest bringing the starter, a salad or a healthy dessert?

Don't be shy, though. If there is anything you don't want to eat, tell the host in advance. If you had an allergy of some sort you would mention it, right?

Some years ago, I had invited my downstairs neighbours for dinner. I had planned and shopped for the meal already. On my way home from work, with just enough time to cook, I bumped into my neighbour, who said: "I did tell you my wife is vegetarian, right?" He hadn't. All panicky, I got in, and opened all the cupboards to check what I could prepare instead of the meal I had planned. Thankfully, I had just enough ingredients to prepare a vegetarian lasagne.

From that moment on, I now make a point of always asking my guests if there is anything they don't eat. You would be surprised at the stuff people come up with when you only ask. I don't eat mint, peppers, raw onions, pork or shellfish, so I make a point of mentioning it when invited out. And since I went sugar free, I add that to the list. No one has ever told me that I'm difficult or stopped inviting me because of it. Even when I climbed Kilimanjaro in the summer of 2018, that was my dietary requirement, and I got separate vegetables every day up the mountain!

Eating out in restaurants is easier than it used to be. You have a menu, and you can always find something healthy to choose from. But more importantly, nearly every restaurant has their menu online. Checking the menu and deciding ahead of time what you're going to eat helps with making better choices. Deciding upfront means that your decision isn't impaired by the level of your hunger when you sit down. It's very similar to going shopping while hungry.

Restaurant portions are way larger than any recommended serving size. Depending on what you order this is true especially for the protein and carbohydrates portion. Going with friends, I would highly recommend that you share a starter and a main, or just have a main. You can always ask to replace the carbohydrate with some extra vegetables, or just order some extra vegetables and not eat the full portion of carbohydrates. Remember that in all restaurants you can talk to the staff about allergies or dislikes.

You can request your food to be different than on the menu. Today it's very common and not frowned upon like it used to be.

Eventually, you shouldn't really be hungry for any dessert. But if you're really desperate for dessert, my tip is to ask for a spoon and just have a teaspoon of someone's else's dessert for the taste. The first two mouthfuls of any food are the ones where you really taste the flavour. After that, you just keep eating not because you're hungry, but because it's there – especially true with dessert.

You will have some pressure from friends trying to convince you to order more, or to order things you don't want to. That pressure generally comes from those who would like to lose weight but haven't succeeded yet. They just want to feel less guilty about their own choices. Others will respect your choices.

Buffets can be tricky! Especially if we start filling our plate from one side of the buffet and walk along continuing to fill it up. You generally end up with a huge amount on your plate or feel that you missed out and go for seconds. Both lead to overeating. So, here's my tip for buffets: before you pick up a plate, walk along the buffet and look at what's on offer. Once you've seen everything, decide and choose what your protein will be, your vegetables and your carbohydrates. Fill your plate, and that's it. Your meal is served, just like at home. And you didn't even have to cook it ;-)

Birthdays, weddings and other celebrations are all part of life, and you will have a few of those throughout the year. How you deal with them comes down to the choices you make. Try to find out what the food will be like and prepare yourself accordingly.

If the birthday party is all crisps and cakes, make sure that you eat a meal before going, and have a few bites of the birthday cake and a few sips of the bubbly to toast the birthday person. At weddings, make sure you eat beforehand. Especially as the real meal is hours away, and the canapés are not always the best choices. It's all about planning and being prepared when it comes to celebrations.

Coffee out is something new-ish. And somehow it has become coffee and cake. There is very little that's healthy to eat in most coffee shops. I would recommend that you enjoy the coffee or tea and just skip the cake. Have you ever looked at the nutritional value of the cakes in coffee shops?

Last year, I was having a cup of tea with my friend Ilana. We met at Starbucks. I was a little early, or she was a little late (I can't remember), and no table was available. So I waited by the counter and took time to have a look at what they served and the nutritional value they offered for each piece of cake, muffin and biscuit. I have to admit that I was shocked. I never realised that those food items contained so many calories, but more importantly such a huge amount of sugar. When my friend arrived, I asked her what she would have chosen had she ordered something. We both agreed that the teacake would be the best option. With 455kcal and 39g of sugar, just under 10 teaspoons, it's shocking. Even if you shared one, you would still eat 5 teaspoons of sugar in half a teacake!!!

Going out for drinks after work is something very common in the UK, especially when you work in London. The expectations are that everyone buys a round of drinks. Which generally means that the larger the group, the more drinks are being bought.

A good tip is to be one of the first ones to buy a round. That way, if you want to cut the night short, you have done your duties. Nurse your drink and don't worry if some drinks are lining up on the table. Once people have had a few, they will just grab a spare one, not realising it was yours.

Although we all know that alcohol is sugar, it's still a part of life and part of social life for many. You can go to the extreme and go teetotal, or you can learn to choose when you want to have a drink, decide upfront how many drinks you will have and, more importantly, match every glass of alcohol you have with a large glass of water.

Helen was ready to give up alcohol during the week. But at weekends she enjoyed going out with her friends and having a few drinks. However, she realised that after a drinking night she really struggled to control her cravings, and often the rest of the weekend ended up with food she hadn't planned to eat.

I gave her a tip to only grab her next drink after downing a large glass of water. After giving it a try, she proudly told me that not only did she cut down on her drinking, but she didn't have an awful hangover the following day, and still managed to enjoy her night out with her friends. None of her friends noticed what she was doing as she was still enjoying some wine.

One tip I would always give anyone when it comes to social life: never arrive anywhere hungry. Try to have a healthy snack an hour to two hours before going out. That way, you won't be tempted by some bread or nibbles if they are on display.

For all situations, the most important thing is the socialising and the relationships with friends, family and colleagues that you're building during those events. It's not about what you eat and how much you drink. You can have as much fun eating a healthy meal and drinking sparkling water as eating a pizza and downing a bottle of wine. This requires a change in mindset for sure. You have the choice. You are in control.

▓ HOLIDAYS

Holidays can be a stressful time for someone on a weight loss journey. No one wants to mess up all the hard work they've done so far.

> *Mike was going away on his yearly holiday to Italy and was very worried. After all, food in Italy is so tasty. The breakfast buffet in the hotel he was staying at was incredible, and what about the gelato? Every year, he used to put on a stone (just over 6kg) over his 10-day holiday in Italy.*

When going on holidays you have three options:
1. Stick to your new way of eating to the letter.
2. Forget about everything, and just eat and drink as much as you want.
3. Make better choices in general, while still enjoying some of the local specialities or some foods and drinks you normally wouldn't have.

I would highly recommend you consider the last option, even when you're on an all- inclusive holiday. All-inclusive doesn't mean you have to eat everything and anything that is being served. It just means that you don't have to worry about paying for your meals and finding a restaurant, as it's all included in your package.

In the same way that at home you would have fresh, unprocessed food, make the same choices while away. Still think of your protein, your vegetables and a little bit of carbohydrate. Do you really have to binge drink every night, or could you have a drink every other night instead, or even just one cocktail or drink a night? If you generally have pastries at breakfast and a dessert with lunch and dinner, rethink that. Do you really need it all? Or could you cut down to once a day? It's not about sticking to your normal plan, but it's about still being in control and making choices.

This is exactly the same when the holiday period arrives, be it Christmas time, Easter, Diwali, Rosh Hashanah till Sukkot, or any other religious holiday period you observe. Those festive periods don't require you to overeat or indulge during all meals and in between the festive days. Plan all your meals ahead of time, knowing that at specific meals you will eat differently to your new norm. Adapt the other meals accordingly.

It's not because the Quality Street box comes out on Christmas day that it has to come out a week before and a week later all day long. Yes, the shops will sell you festive goodies for weeks and months ahead of time. Christmas food is in the shops now from the end of August trying to tempt you, and Easter eggs come out the day after Christmas. That doesn't mean you have to buy this food then, let alone eat it!

As our lives have become busier and more social, here is a great tip. We all have 52 weeks in a year. If you're lucky you might be going away on holidays for 2-4 weeks a year. Add some long weekends, birthdays, weddings and special occasions. Does that add up to about 6 weeks? Can you really mess up the focused and on-plan work you're doing over 46 weeks in the space of 6 weeks (spread out over the year)? You would really have to go totally overboard to be able to do that. So, when going away and attending special events, feel free to relax a little. It's a special time after all.

Summary:

Understanding what you're eating and drinking and how it affects your weight and health is very important.

Eating natural, nutrition-rich food in the right proportions is key.

You can't separate health and weight loss. If you eat badly, your health will suffer. If you don't feel well, you will be tempted to comfort eat with unhealthy foods.

Eating for health might not be your first priority, but it should be. It has a direct effect on your weight loss.

STEP 4
EXERCISE AND ACTIVITY

What is the best exercise for weight loss?
What exercises should I do to get rid of my bingo wings?
I hate my thighs... how can I reduce my flabby thighs?
What about my muffin top? How many sit-ups do I really need to do every day to get rid of it?

Frequent questions I'm asked when people find out that I'm a personal trainer. Let me start by saying that there is no right or wrong exercise. And there is no better or worse one either. It's about finding something that you enjoy doing.

If you were to join an exercise programme today and, although you would expect the first few sessions to be hard, hated every moment of it, how long do you think you could keep consistent with it? What would happen at every opportunity you could find a way to get out of going? A planned event, a last-minute call from your friends to go out, a cold or rainy day? If you're like most of us, any excuse will be the one to use to get out of going. But if you were to enjoy the activity and look forward to going to it on a weekly basis or more? How likely would you be then to skip a session?

A client of mine started her 12-week programme with me a few years ago. She attended all her sessions, but I could see and feel that she hated coming. She just wasn't enjoying it. There were exercises she didn't want to do, and others she did reluctantly.

We sat down one day after the session, and I told her I didn't feel the programme was actually right for her. I asked her if there was any other type of exercise that she would enjoy doing, knowing that she hadn't been active for quite some years. I saw a flicker in her eyes when she told me that her dream was to go to ballroom dancing classes. We parted ways very amicably, and she's been dancing ever since and loving every moment of it.

Today, when we talk about exercise, one of the first images that comes to mind for most is the gym, or people running in the local park. But do we really need to go to the gym to exercise? Take my client above… her dance sessions weren't held in the gym.

These days, I don't train my clients in a gym. When I started my personal trainer career I did home visits, and brought some portable equipment with me, while training other clients in the park. The last few years I've been hiring a space out, as I wanted to be able to see more clients, as well as do some small group sessions.

Exercise can be done anywhere: at home, outdoors, at an exercise class in a hall, at the gym or at a leisure centre. It really doesn't matter where you're doing the exercise, as long as you do the following 4 types of things: movement, cardiovascular exercise, strength training, plus mobility, flexibility and stretching.

■ MOVEMENT

Our bodies are meant to move! And movement doesn't mean exercise. It's only our culture and environment that make us sedentary. And with being sedentary comes dormant muscles, imbalances, stiffness, aches and pains.

How many hours a day do you sit at work, at home or during your commute? All that sitting affects your muscles, your joints, your lung capacity, your lymphatic system and your heart health.

So, let's start by looking at how you can add more movement throughout your day and week. And I'm not talking about your exercise class. I'm talking about just being more active and moving more during the day.

> Could you walk your kids to school?
> Could you walk to work, or walk part of the way?
> Could you walk to the shops for small purchases?
> Could you get up every hour and move around?
> Could you take the stairs?
> If you're on a high floor, how about just walking up some of them?

I can't recall the name of the TV programme I watched some years ago, but they put some electrodes to monitor activity and metabolism rate onto an office worker and a waitress. As expected, the waitress's readings were much higher than the office worker's, as she was moving around all day long. To check what would happen to his metabolism if he were moving more, they asked that for a week he walked part way to work, got up and paced around while on the phone, took the stairs, and walked out at lunchtime to eat his lunch instead of eating at his desk. His activity levels and metabolism rate went right up.

If you have a faster metabolism you burn more calories, hence over time it's easier to lose more weight (at least if you don't start eating more).

My client Nima started a new job at a new school. The building was much larger than at her previous school. Her classroom was one of the furthest away from the staffroom, and on the 3rd floor. Naturally, she had to walk more and climb many more steps every day. A month after starting her new job, at her monthly tracking session, even without changing anything else the results of being more active during the daytime showed, both on the scales and in the measurements.

The nice thing about being more active and moving more is that nearly anyone at any age can do it.

Exercise

Think about 3 ways that you can increase your movement and be more active during the day.

■ CARDIOVASCULAR VS STRENGTH TRAINING

In my first few months as a personal trainer, I worked on the gym floor. A girl came up to me and told me that she was in the process of losing weight. She was on a strict diet, and she was doing loads of cardiovascular exercise. She was aiming to lose 3 stone. And when she'd achieved that, she would sign up for some sessions with me to get herself toned. Somehow, she never got to her goal, and after a month I never saw her at the gym again.

There are so many options out there when it comes to exercise. From traditional cardiovascular exercise and strength or weight training to a mixture of both through high intensity interval training (HIIT).

We have already discussed the fact that doing something you like is important. Into what category does what you enjoy doing fall?

For health reasons, as well as for weight loss reasons, it is important to do both cardiovascular and strength training. But it doesn't have to be mixed in the same session, and it doesn't mean you have to go to a specific class or follow a specific programme.

Cardiovascular exercise is an important type of exercise. While doing it, your heart rate goes up, and as your heart is a muscle, it's being worked. With consistency, frequency and persistency, your heart will allow you to go faster, further and for a longer period of time, and your heart will get stronger along the way.

When it comes to weight loss, cardiovascular exercise is great, as you burn calories and speed up your metabolism while you're exercising. So, if you are going for a 30-minute fast walk, you will speed up your metabolism and burn calories for approximately 30 minutes.

Please ignore any calorie data you get from your phone, apps, Fitbit, cardio machine or any other device that is available to non-athletes like us. The data you get on how many calories you've burned is massively overestimated.

Strength training or weight training is as important as cardiovascular exercise for health and weight loss purposes. Many women shy away from strength or weight training because they worry that they will bulk up. If that's you, then don't worry – you won't bulk up. Unless you start lifting heavy weights, eating a huge amount of protein and adding some testosterone (male hormones), you won't be bulking up. Naturally we're not made to bulk up.

However, our muscles, and our bones as we age, need strength training. This can be done using your body weight only, or by adding weights from light to heavy. In the same way that consistency, frequency and persistency help to get your cardiovascular system up, the same counts for your muscle strength.

It is important to remember to train all body parts, to vary your exercises regularly, and to increase the load to keep your muscles reacting to your effort. I would highly recommend that you take up a few sessions with a personal trainer to show you the correct technique for strength training. Using too heavy weights or not having the correct posture during the exercise can easily lead to injuries.

The great thing with strength training is that, depending on the intensity of the session, your metabolism will be heightened for up to 48 hours after your workout. This is due to the fact that as you perform the exercises, you are causing micro-tears to your muscle fibres. This is needed to build stronger muscle mass. It takes up to 48 hours for your muscles to repair. During that time, your metabolism will be working harder than normal, and you will often experience DOMS (delayed onset muscle soreness). It's also one of the reasons why it's not advised to work the same muscles two days in a row.

So I would encourage you not to do strength training on consecutive days, unless you separate body parts. Lower body one day, upper body the following day, for instance, or if you are willing to learn more about how the muscles work, you could train opposite muscle groups on alternate days.

You might have heard of HIIT training, which is a combination of strength training and cardiovascular training. Generally, you alternate between the two, so that you perform your strength exercises while having a heightened heart rate from the cardiovascular exercise. It's a great way of training if you are short of time. But as the pace is higher, and you're trying to recover from your cardio exercise, the correct form of the strength exercise is often forgotten. Which can lead to injuries. If you're a beginner to exercise, I would not recommend HIIT training.

Ever been to an exercise class where you're working really hard for 45 minutes with minimal breaks, you're never too sure you're doing the exercises correctly, or are still busy with one exercise when the teacher has already started on the next one?

Unfortunately, as classes are generally large, many people get injured due to not focusing on technique, but just focusing on keeping up with the class.

If you decide to have a longer session and combine your cardiovascular exercise with your strength training without it being in HIIT format, I would suggest that you do a short warm-up, then perform your strength training, and then move onto your cardiovascular exercise. Most people I see do it the other way around. There are two reasons for following my method:

1. As I already mentioned, it's important to keep good form when it comes to strength training. By doing your cardiovascular exercise first, you deplete your muscles of glycogen, which then means that you have limited strength left for your strength training.
2. When doing your strength training first, you also deplete your glycogen levels, hence when doing your cardiovascular exercise you are forced to dig into your fat reserves for energy purposes.

If you're short of time, there is still plenty you can do. Use your time wisely. Working with my clients, I encourage them to use "dead" time to do something. Waiting for the kettle to boil? How about doing some press-ups against the kitchen counter, performing some squats or lunges, or just running on the spot? Stand on one leg while brushing your teeth in the mornings and on the other one in the evenings.

What other "dead" times could you use to do some exercise when you're short of time?

Of course, doing a full session is more beneficial. But when you're short of time… **something is better than nothing.**

▓ MOBILITY, FLEXIBILITY AND STRETCHING

One thing most of us forget when we think of exercise is mobility, flexibility and stretching. I can't stress the importance of those enough, especially as we age.

As kids, during PE, we barely did any. No warm-up, no mobilisation – we just went straight into the class, and there were no stretches at the end. Most of us ran around the playground during break time. As adults, we generally do our exercise, come home and, after a shower, just get on with our lives. Most of our workouts do not include any warm-up or proper cool down and stretches.

If you haven't done any specific mobility, flexibility and stretching exercises so far, then I highly recommend you start looking at integrating them into your routine as of today. Find a stretch, Pilates, yoga or tai chi class. A good book I would recommend is one called *Stretching* by Bob Anderson. Learn how to use a foam roller and a lacrosse ball to relieve tension. Look up myofascial release – a great way to self- massage and (re)gain some mobility.

Ideally, after a day being sedentary, it would be great to do a 5-10 minute routine at the end of the day. Find a soft carpet or invest in a mat. And incorporate stretches at the end of every workout you're doing. As with any other activity, the more consistent you become, the more benefit you will get out of it. It's also a great way to reduce your stress levels.

▓ HOW MUCH EXERCISE, HOW OFTEN AND FOR HOW LONG?

The NHS (https://www.nhs.uk/live-well/exercise/) recommends the following. To stay healthy, adults aged 19 to 64 should try to be active daily and should do:

at least 150 minutes of moderate aerobic activity such as cycling or brisk walking every week and strength exercises on 2 or more days a week that work all the major muscles (legs, hips, back, abdomen, chest, shoulders and arms)

or

75 minutes of vigorous aerobic activity such as running or a game of singles tennis every week and strength exercises on 2 or more days a week that work all the major muscles (legs, hips, back, abdomen, chest, shoulders and arms)

or

a mix of moderate and vigorous aerobic activity every week – for example, 2 x 30-minute runs plus 30 minutes of brisk walking equates to 150 minutes of moderate aerobic activity and strength exercises on 2 or more days a week that work all the major muscles (legs, hips, back, abdomen, chest, shoulders and arms)

A good rule is that 1 minute of vigorous activity provides the same health benefits as 2 minutes of moderate activity. One way to do your recommended 150 minutes of weekly physical activity is to do 30 minutes on 5 days every week.

All adults should also break up long periods of sitting with light activity. Moderate activity will raise your heart rate and make you breathe faster and feel warmer. One way to tell if you're working at a moderate level is if you can still talk, but you can't sing the words to a song. Vigorous activity makes you breathe hard and fast. If you're working at this level, you won't be able to say more than a few words without pausing for breath.

The government recommendations are very confusing, leaving everyone guessing. How much exercise does one really have to do to lose weight?

On my 12-week programmes, I see my clients twice a week for an hour of full body strength training, and they get great results with that. I obviously recommend being active and moving as much as possible, and potentially doing some other form of exercise on the other days.

Could you do more? Yes, you definitely could. But remember not to work out the same muscle part two days in a row. If you worked hard, these muscles need a rest to recover.

Could you be doing too much? Yes, you definitely could. Working out too much, especially when you are super busy or run down, can be a stressor to your body. I mentioned earlier that stress is a cause of too much cortisol release. And that can prevent you from losing weight. Which in turn will cause you more stress as you just won't understand why you're not ditching those pounds.

It's really a bit of trial and error to find the right balance for you when it comes to exercise. As you get fitter and stronger, you will probably need to change what exercise you're doing and how you're doing it if you want to continue to see progress. Very similar to how much food to eat daily as you lose weight.

How long every session needs to be is a great question. A session can be anything from 5 minutes up to 90 minutes long. Yes, 5 minutes is sometimes enough, especially when you're short of time. Ever tried to run up and down the stairs for 5 minutes non-stop? Try it and see how you feel ;-)

In the Habits step, we discussed planning and scheduling your exercise sessions in the diary. There will be days when things don't go to plan and you have to skip your planned session. On those days, try to do something for 5 minutes only.

Something is always better than nothing!

Yes, 5 minutes is better than skipping your session altogether. And it can be anything – even dancing like a lunatic around your lounge. The important thing is to be consistent with your exercise. Going flat out for a few days, and then stopping for 2 weeks because you're too busy, won't give you the results you want. Which is why even short workouts regularly are highly recommended if you struggle with time or a routine.

When I worked in the corporate world, I never knew where I would be as I was travelling so much. When I was home, I tried to go to the gym. If I hadn't booked a session with a personal trainer, all the excuses on earth why not to go came up. But I wasn't home enough to have regular sessions. Every session with the trainer was hard and, because I wasn't consistent due to being away, I didn't progress in strength, in fitness or in weight loss. It got very frustrating, and that eventually led to many unused gym memberships.

Had I known at the time that a 5-10 minute workout in my hotel room would have kept me on track in between the sessions when I was home, I'm sure I would have achieved the results I wanted, albeit more slowly. I wouldn't have given up – asking myself what the point was.

It's not enough to just exercise full on for a few days and then stop. It's the consistency and frequency that will give you the results you want.

■ TIMING OF EXERCISE

I'm often asked if it's best to work out first thing in the morning, as your body is then burning more calories throughout the day. And what about working out before breakfast, when your glycogen reserves are low after fasting through the night, and you then automatically burn fat?

> *I'm not a morning person. I really struggle to get out of bed in the mornings and to be awake and focused first thing. I was the kid that was late for school every morning. On the good days, I sneaked in just as the bell was ringing. Having cut out sugar has definitely helped me to get out of bed more easily and to be a little more awake first thing. But it still takes me about 1-2 hours to be fully focused. When working out, that focus makes a huge difference. Doing the same workout from mid-morning onwards, I can achieve much more and push much harder than if I do it first thing. So, no matter what anyone says, having a better workout from mid-morning onwards will be better for me for long-term results and adherence.*

Listen to your body, try different options, and see what works best for you. Most importantly, see when you can fit your workouts better into your schedule. If you're not a morning person and you schedule your workouts at 6 a.m. you most probably will go a couple of times, then skip your workouts on the mornings you struggle to get out of bed.

Remember, consistency is the most important thing! Does it always have to be at the same time each week? There are some arguments for and against. Stay flexible. **A workout done is better than one not done, no matter what time of day.**

If you do work out in the evenings, just make sure you have enough time to properly cool down before going to sleep. Depending on the intensity of your workout, this can take a little longer. A nice, relaxing bath with some Epsom salts can definitely help to speed things up.

Do schedule your workouts in your diary, just like any other meeting or activity. If it's not in the diary, the chances of skipping it are much higher. Remember that if your schedule changes, 5 minutes is better than nothing.

Exercise

What exercise do I enjoy doing?
What days and times can I realistically commit to exercise?
What exercise would I love to learn or get better at?
Where can I find a class or a teacher to help me with it?

■ FOOD BEFORE AND AFTER EXERCISE

Should you eat before your workout?
What should you eat?
How long before?
Do you need an energy drink during your workout?
What about after?

All good questions!

If you're training for a specific event or you're an athlete, then my answer would be very different to what I'm going to say now. If your goal is to lose weight, and therefore exercise is part of your weight loss regime and also for maintenance afterwards, then my advice would be as follows:

Don't worry too much about timings. Stick to your regular eating habits as on any other day.

If you had your meal quite a few hours before your workout, you can have a snack 1-2 hours before. Let's say you tend to work out after work around 6 p.m., and you had your lunch at 1 p.m., have a snack around 4:30-5 p.m.

If you are an early morning workout person, and don't fancy waking up even earlier, then a small snack 30-45 minutes before could work, but I suggest you try and see what works for you. You might feel you're still digesting your snack, and it might be best to just have your workout and come back for your regular breakfast.

After your workout, make sure you focus on eating some protein, even if you're only having a snack again, depending on the time of day. For anything longer than a 2-hour workout, I would start thinking about how to include some snack or a home-made energy drink. For any regular workout up to 90 minutes, plain water is perfectly fine to hydrate during your session. No need to guzzle on an energy drink.

One thing to remember, no matter what exercise you do and how much: **you can't out-train a bad diet!** Your eating habits are as important as your exercise if you want to achieve weight loss. Don't think that because you had a workout you can now eat that bar of chocolate!

▨ NO PAIN, NO GAIN

Tanya signed up to work with me on my 1:1 programme. We had our first session, and she really enjoyed it. She came back for her second session and told me that it was the first time she had actually had a hard workout but wasn't crippled for 10 days afterwards. Her previous experiences with personal trainers were short-lived, as she had to keep on cancelling her sessions due to massive soreness.

If you want to see change, you have to work out just outside your comfort zone during most sessions. Suffering from DOMS – delayed onset muscle soreness – is normal. But it shouldn't be crippling. The stiffness (DOMS) you feel is because your muscles have been worked out just outside their comfort zone, you've torn some muscle fibres (micro-tears, so don't worry about them) and now your muscles need time and good healthy protein to rebuild stronger than before. As mentioned earlier, that period of time only takes up to 48 hours. If it takes more time to recover, it means you pushed way too hard.

If a trainer tells you that no pain, no gain is part of the deal, then run! We've already said that consistency and frequency are key. If you can't stick to it due to working out too hard, you will never achieve the results you want.

■ INCH LOSS VS WEIGHT LOSS

"Muscles weigh more than fat."
"When you lift weights, you transform fat into muscle."

I would be a millionaire if I collected £1 each time I heard those statements. I used to think similarly until I studied anatomy as part of my personal trainer course.

1kg of muscle weighs exactly the same as 1kg of fat. And you can't transform fat into muscle. They're totally different in structure, so you can't turn one into the other.

When you work out, mixing all types of exercises – cardiovascular and strength – you burn calories and build muscle mass. Both in turn will burn fat. The space 1kg of muscle takes is way less than the space taken up by 1kg of fat. So, if you lose inches by building more muscle mass, it means that you have lost fat.

One of the things I do with my clients at their tracking session every 4 weeks is a weigh-in, as well as measurement tracking. Some months you will see a decrease in both weight and measurements, and sometimes the scales might not have budged much, but the measurements are showing progress. Another reason why it's not all about the scales!

For health reasons, inch loss is much more important than the number on the scales. Losing fat, especially around the middle, is a good indicator of getting healthier. Fat pressing on your internal organs is not healthy and is an associated risk factor for many diseases.

If you could choose only one of the following, what would you choose? Fitting into smaller-sized clothes and looking trim, fit and strong, or being lighter and flabby?

Summary:

Exercise and movement are as important for health reasons as they are for weight loss. The combination of movement, cardiovascular and strength training, as well as mobility, is crucial.

Consistency and frequency are key to seeing results. Something is always better than nothing. Even 5 minutes is better than just skipping exercise altogether when short of time.

Exercise might not always show results on the scales, but often will do on the tape measure. Inch loss is more important for health reasons than weight.

One can't out-train a bad diet.

STEP 5
SLEEP AND STRESS

As a result of our busy lives, our lifestyle and technology, sleep has taken a massive hit and has become something that is regarded as an essential evil, taking us away from our days. Which is why in today's world we only sleep a minimum amount of hours to get us through all we have to do, often aided by huge quantities of caffeine to keep us going.

We currently live in a sleep-deprived society, and in research done by Rand Europe in 2016, lack of sleep cost the UK economy £40 billion a year, or 200,000 working days. The US was no better off with a loss of £328 billion a year, or 1.2 million working days.

How many "duvet" days have you taken or considered taking over the past few years? The effect of lack of sleep is not just about the cost to society. It has a massive effect on our health, our family life, our environment and, as a result, on our weight.

Another result of our busy lives and everything around them is the increase in stress levels. As a result, there is a huge increase in people struggling with mental health issues such as anxiety and depression. Stress is often ignored due to it being perceived as people not being able to cope and being weak.

The amount of people who are being prescribed antidepressants is on the increase year after year. The number of prescriptions for antidepressants in England has almost doubled in the past decade, new figures have shown.

The March 2019 edition of the British Medical Journal, with data from NHS Digital shows that 70.9 million prescriptions for antidepressants were given out in 2018, compared with 36 million in 2008. The number has been steadily increasing year-on-year, with 64.7 million given out in 2016 and 67.5 million prescribed in 2017. (BMJ 2019;364: l1508) Those numbers only include prescriptions given out by NHS England. They exclude those given out in hospitals or private prescriptions, and they do not include the rest of the UK!

The level of stress we're under and our inability to cope has a major effect on our health, our environment and, as a result, our weight. So how exactly are these related to our weight loss journey and what can we do to use sleep and stress to our advantage?

▓ SLEEP

When I talk to friends about sleep, I often get the proud response that they manage very well on 5 hours a night and don't feel they need more. They go to bed late, and they wake up super early to be able to achieve more. But do they really?

How many hours do you currently sleep at night? It's not just about the number of hours, but also about the quality of your sleep. Do you feel rested when you get up in the morning?

Sleep is an essential part of a weight loss journey on many levels. During our sleep, the body recovers from the past day, and prepares itself for the day ahead. While we sleep, our blood pressure drops, our muscles relax, our blood sugar levels balance, the blood supply to our muscle increases, tissue growth and repair occur, energy is restored, hormones are released and replenished, energy is provided to the brain and the body, the immune system is strengthened, and a few other processes are happening.

We've already seen in the hormone chapter that the hunger and satiety hormones, ghrelin and leptin, are affected by lack of sleep. As well as hormones being affected and working from within to push us to eat more, lack of sleep also affects our focus and judgment and makes it harder to make healthy food choices. We're very likely to grab sugary food for a quick energy burst, or a stimulant like caffeine to keep us going. Lack of energy makes it harder to cook from scratch when it takes more time and effort than getting a takeaway. And the last thing you feel like doing is exercising. After all, you're already tired!

I'm sure you've heard it before… we do need 7-8 hours of sleep a night. And that doesn't mean 7-8 hours in bed. Add half an hour to that so as to get the full time of quality sleep. Having broken sleep for 7-8 hours is not the same as having 7-8 hours of uninterrupted sleep. Knowing all this, let's see how we can improve our sleep quantity and quality.

To be able to have a good night's sleep, it's important to wind down about 1 hour before bedtime. Some might say longer, but let's stay realistic and keep it to 1 hour. The winding down is what we're going to call a bedtime routine.

Do you remember your bedtime routine as a child? Or your own children's bedtime routine? Dinner, bath, story time, cuddles, and off to bed. All activities to help children wind down and go to sleep more easily.

We as adults need exactly the same!

In an ideal world, you'd go to sleep every night at the same time, and you'd wake up every morning at the same time. Try to be as close to that as possible so as not to disturb your natural body clock, or what's called a circadian clock. Your bedtime routine should start with disconnecting from all electronic devices. It's easier said than done but, over a period of a few weeks, build up to it.

Until a few years ago, I used to aimlessly scroll through social media once in bed. I found it relaxing, or so I thought. I could easily spend 30-45 minutes on my phone every night. And it was the first thing I picked up in the morning for another 30-45 minutes. I didn't want to miss out on anything – FOMO!

I've never been much of a morning person, but every morning I woke up exhausted. As I was meeting with a few other health professionals, we discussed how we could improve our productivity. I mentioned that morning times weren't great for me. My friend Alison pointed out that due to my "phone habits", at the end of the week I had lost a whole night's sleep – 7-8 hours!!!! That was a massive eye-opener for me. I hadn't thought about it like that. A whole night's sleep!

Since then, unless in emergency situations, my phone has been left far away from my bed. I still use it as my alarm clock, which then means I have to get out of bed and be up to switch it off. The good thing is that I've started tackling the pile of books I had amassed over the years and never had time to read.

Pick up a book and read instead. Ideally a paper book, or an e-reader that doesn't emit any blue light. The blue light and radiation that electronic devices emit is a brainwave activator. Before bedtime, you want something calming to help you to fall asleep more easily. Listen to relaxing music if you don't like the silence. Dim your lights if you can. Engage in some relaxation activities for 5-30 minutes (we'll go through some in the stress chapter). Go to bed.

It's important that your bedroom has the right temperature and is as dark as possible, and as quiet as possible. We sleep best in a cool room. So, if you have central heating on in the house, make sure it goes off as you start your bedtime routine, so that your bedroom has cooled down in time for sleep time. You might think that falling asleep with a TV on is the right thing to do, but the constant noise just keeps your brain awake and prevents you from gaining quality sleep.

If for whatever reason you can't fall asleep or you wake up and can't get back to sleep, don't toss and turn in bed. Get out of bed, and out of the bedroom. Go and read something, or do some breathing exercises in a different room, but don't reach out to electronic devices! When you're ready to sleep again, get back into bed.

If you eat well, exercise well, and relax well, you will see a big improvement in your sleeping patterns. And vice versa. In the same way that identity plays a role in weight loss, it also plays a role in sleep.

Robert had been struggling with his sleep for years. Some days he couldn't fall asleep for hours and on others he woke up a few hours later and couldn't fall asleep again. He defined himself as an insomniac. He had been tossing and turning in bed, and eventually resorted to scrolling on his phone watching YouTube videos. He was always tired, ate lots of processed food, drank jugs of coffee, and suffered with regular migraines.

He had tried lots of different things such as having a bath before bedtime, plus lots of different pills and herbal remedies. He dabbled a little into white noise and meditation. Nothing seemed to help.

Changing his eating habits, reducing his caffeine intake, getting him to exercise more and to have a bedtime routine massively improved his sleep, both in time and quality. It didn't happen overnight, though. It was a process that took about 10 weeks before seeing improvements, and a few more months before he really felt a big difference.

The problem with most people who struggle with sleep is that they try something for a few days or a week, and if it doesn't work, they stop. Very similar to diets and magic diet pills.

If you work in a job with changing shifts, or doing the night shift, it's tricky, because you are fighting against your circadian clock. Try to have as much of a routine as you possibly can. And make sure that if your sleep is during daytime, you definitely have black-out blinds and a fully dark room.

Having a new-born baby up to the time that they're sleeping through the night is another reason that can make having your full 7-8 hours' sleep or uninterrupted sleep tricky. Try to sleep when your little one does, or at least as much as possible. It's not going to be perfect. You will be tired. Just don't make it harder on yourself by reaching out to coffee or processed and sugary foods. Long term, it will make getting back to a good routine much harder.

Unless you work split shifts or have a small baby you might think that having a long nap at the weekend is enough to catch up on lost sleep. It isn't, unfortunately. Having a nap is a great way to reduce stress, but it doesn't compensate for lack of sleep every night. It might help if you had one bad night, but not when you suffer from consistent sleep deprivation. For some it's also important to note that when you have a nap in the afternoon it may lead to less sleep or a lower quality of sleep at night.

Exercise

Write out your bedtime routine.

■ STRESS

When we think about traditional diets and weight loss, our stress levels immediately go up. The associations we make with the words dieting, diets and weight loss are so negative. The feelings that come up are so negative. It's no surprise that we're getting stressed and overwhelmed just by thinking about weight loss.

Unless you implement the steps outlined in this book, it's going to stay stressful. Being stressed generally leads to making unhealthy choices food and drink-wise. It is therefore important to understand what causes us stress and to have some techniques to reduce it.

We all have cortisol, the stress hormone, in our body. We need to have it – otherwise we would barely move. Naturally, the levels of cortisol are higher in the morning, and go down as the day goes by and we're getting ready for a good night's sleep. However, our natural system is affected by everything going on during our day.

I'd like you to start noticing how events happening throughout your day affect you. From the kids not getting dressed quickly enough, or being grumpy at breakfast, to a traffic jam on the school run, no seat on public transport, a few emails that require you to do unplanned work, an unscheduled meeting that affects your lunch break, skipping meals because you're too busy, an argument with someone, your internet going down, a call from school to pick up your ill child, your elderly parent not being well, a really hard workout, too much exercise... the list is endless!

And then there are longer-term stresses such as uncertainty at work, redundancy, job hunting, going through a divorce, having a little baby in the house or even a puppy, caring for an ill friend or relative, and more. How do these events affect you? How do you react to them?

Every time you react, you are spiking your cortisol levels. The big question is, by how much? How intense is your reaction, and how quickly do you calm down? When we're stressed, our nervous system is on alert. The nervous system is made up of 2 main divisions: the somatic or voluntary system and the autonomic or involuntary system.

The somatic system is used when you consciously do something. Let's say you reach out to a cup of tea – your brain gives out a conscious signal to muscles and nerves to reach out and get hold of your cup of tea.

Your autonomic system is taking care of all the things we don't even think of. Breathing, digestion, heart pumping away, your pupil responses to light changes, etc. We're not even aware of those.

The autonomic system is then divided into two. The sympathetic nervous system releases cortisol when under stress, causes us to breathe faster, our heart to pump faster, to sweat more, get more focused, and it internally takes us away from normal digestion and a few other normal activities that happen in the background. All that to give some much-needed resource to respond to our stress level. The parasympathetic nervous system is what calms us down and restores our normal functioning. It lowers our heart rate to normal again, calms our breathing, gets us to digest our food again, and more.

The problem is not short bursts of stress. The problem occurs when we stay stressed for a prolonged time. And a prolonged time is anything longer than half an hour to an hour. If our digestive system is impaired on a regular basis because our sympathetic nervous system needs resources to fight a stressful situation then we don't break down our food properly, we don't ingest valuable nutrients, we feel bloated, sluggish and potentially even get constipated. Over time, this can lead to IBS, leaky gut and other digestive disorders. Having a healthy gut is crucial for weight loss, the immune system, and other vital systems which all affect the way we act and react to life situations including food choices.

So we absolutely need to reduce our stress levels on a daily basis. If you've been living under stress for a long time, you won't even consider yourself as being stressed. But adopting some of the following techniques will make a big difference in your life, even if right now you don't feel like they will.

The first thing I want you to do is to schedule 5-20 minutes a day as "me-time". It doesn't have to be at the same time every day, as long as it happens every day. Yes, be selfish for 5-20 minutes a day. It will have a positive ripple effect on everyone around you. You can't pour from an empty jug. So start filling that jug again.

Now what to do during those 5-20 minutes is totally up to you. An activity that you find relaxing and helps you to switch off from your daily life. When I ask my clients what they enjoy doing as relaxation activities, I often get a blank stare. It's often an effort to come up with something, because it hasn't been a subject that has been discussed or contemplated in a long time, if ever.

So here are some ideas: a bath, meditation, a walk in the fresh air, breathing exercises, stretches, listening to some calming music, reading a book, writing a gratitude journal, writing a book, drawing, colouring, singing, watching the sunset, sitting on a bench and watching the sea, having a facial, going for a massage… even watching TV would work as long as it's not a subject that gets you all wound up. There are plenty more!

Once you start thinking and digging, I'm sure you can come up with many more activities that you find relaxing. Just don't choose to sit on the sofa with a glass of wine to "unwind". Alcohol is a stress to the body as it's a stimulant.

Make sure those 5-20 minutes are uninterrupted. No kids, no partners, no phone calls, no emails... nothing. Just you and your activity.

Exercise

Write down all the activities you find relaxing.

Conclusion

Now you know what it takes to lose weight once and for all and to lead a healthy lifestyle, all while leading a busy life.

You can't focus on diet and exercise alone. It's not enough, and it just won't work. At least not for long-term results. You have to focus on all 5 steps for that.

It's about first and foremost being very clear about your why, and finding one that is meaningful enough to lead you to action and sustain it.

Then it's about realising that losing weight is a journey – a learning curve – where perfection doesn't have a place.

It's about making a plan – your plan – that works for you and can fit into your life. That plan will break down every subject covered in the book into smaller bite-sized chunks. You will then choose 1-2 chunks from each step that you feel confident to take on. Once those chunks become your new norm, you can move on to the next few.

You now understand why your plan will not be the same as someone else's plan, which is why following box-standard diets has not worked for you in the past. Especially since those diets didn't include any guidance on mindset, habits, sleep or stress, and often had contradictory information about exercise.

You are ready for your life to change. You can't expect the results you want by hanging onto your current mindset and the habits that don't benefit you. You won't be the same person you have been so far. You will become a better and more positive version of yourself. You will be releasing the real you!

Be kind to yourself, take time for yourself, make yourself and your health a priority, and learn about yourself every day. Be patient. It's the only way you will become the person you deep down want to be.

Taking that time is not being selfish. A happier, more confident and fulfilled you will have a ripple effect on everything you do, and on everyone around you.

Download the exercises in the book and complete them. Here's the link again:
https://anneiarchy.com/5-simple-steps-companion-sheets/

Track your progress, and review and analyse what's going on for you regularly.

It's totally OK to reach out and ask for help. You don't have to be superhuman and do it all alone.

Find a community of supportive like-minded people who have your back. I'm inviting you to join my Facebook community *It's Not About the Scales.*

If you are ready to take action, and feel that you could benefit from professional guidance, then reach out and let's have a chat about how I can help you – whether face-to-face locally in North London, through some of my workshops and events, or via my online programme, *Slimmer U Club.*

You can do it! I believe in you!!

About the Author

Anne Iarchy is a successful weight loss and healthy lifestyle coach.

After struggling with her own weight and confidence issues while working in the corporate world, it is now her mission to help self-employed women break free from the diet trap, and understand why they are stuck. More importantly, Anne wants to show women what they need to put in place to regain their confidence, self-esteem, happiness, health and energy to perform at their best.

As a busy professional she found it nearly impossible to live a healthy lifestyle, and in addition, couldn't find anyone to help her with the struggles of regular work travel as well as trying to enjoy a social and family life.

Her weight and health severely dented her confidence and self-esteem.

After qualifying as a personal trainer in 2007, in 2010 she eventually made a big career change from sales director in an IT security company to setting up her own business in the health, weight loss and wellbeing field.

Her own experience and work with clients over the past 10 years has helped her build and shape her personal 5 step system.

Anne is passionate about human behaviour, habit change, nutrition, and how food manufacturers produce and package food to make us both eat and buy more.

In her spare time, she loves the outdoors, golf, swimming and spinning.

Every year, Anne participates in a charity challenge and over the years she has cycled and walked London to Brighton, climbed Kilimanjaro, swam 22 miles over 12 weeks and 5km non-stop, and ran the London Marathon. In addition, she volunteers with several charities and project, including mentoring low-level first-time offenders.

If you would like to get in touch with Anne, please email her on anne@anneiarchy.com or find her on Facebook, Twitter or Instagram.

Acknowledgements

This book would not have happened without all the clients I've been working with over the past 10 years.

I've learned so much from each and everyone of them. It's their struggles and problems that have pushed me to learn, research, explore, trial, improve and grow. Working with them eventually culminated into developing my 5 simple steps system.

Secondly, I'd like to thank my parents, brother, sister-in-law, my gorgeous nieces, and my grandmother who unfortunately isn't with us anymore. They've been supportive of me throughout, no matter what crazy idea I've come up with over the years. And I know my grandmother would be very proud of me right now for writing this book.

My two besties, Rakhee Shah and Lucy Howe have pushed me over the years we've known each other to show up as my best self. They've been my cheerleaders during good and bad times and I'm very grateful for that.

Writing a book had been on my bucket list for a few years now. I just had no clue how to even start the process. Shaa Wasmund MBE and Lucy McCarraher showed me how to structure and write my book.

A big thank you to Brenda Dempsey who introduced me to the team at Filament Publishing: Chris Day, Olivia Eisinger, Zara Thatcher and their teams.

You've made publishing the book easy, even if at some point I didn't think we'd ever agree on a front cover and title!

Bibliography

■ BOOKS

Dr Rangan Chatterjee, *The Stress Solution*, Penguin Life, 2018

Pete Cohen, *Shut the Duck Up!*, Filament Publishing, 2015

Charles Duhigg, *The Power of Habit*, Random House Books, 2013

Benjamin Hardy, *Willpower Doesn't Work*, Piatkus, 2018

■ MAGAZINES AND JOURNALS

British Medical Journal – various